'A NECESSITY AMONG US'

DAVID GAGAN

'A Necessity Among Us'
The Owen Sound General
and Marine Hospital 1891–1985

Published for Grey Bruce Regional Health Centre
BY UNIVERSITY OF TORONTO PRESS
Toronto Buffalo London

© University of Toronto Press 1990
Toronto Buffalo London
Printed in Canada

ISBN 0-8020-3462-4

Printed on acid-free paper

---

**Canadian Cataloguing in Publication Data**

Gagan, David, 1940–
  A necessity among us

ISBN 0-8020-3462-4

1. Owen Sound General and Marine Hospital –
History. 2. Hospitals – Ontario – Owen Sound –
History. I. Grey Bruce Regional Health Centre.
II. Title.

RA983.093093 1990    362.1'1'0971318    C90-093850-1

*For my mother and in memory of my father*

# Contents

LIST OF ILLUSTRATIONS / ix

PREFACE / xi

1 'A Great Opportunity of Doing Good': Founding the G&M, 1885–93 / 3

2 'A Public Utility': The Emergence of the Modern Hospital, 1893–1914 / 28

3 'Once a Patient, Always a Booster': Standardization and Stability, 1914–29 / 57

4 'Sickness Is an Expensive Luxury': Depression, War, and the Crisis of Health Care, 1930–49 / 84

5 'What Can a Drowning Man Afford for a Life Jacket?' The Politics of Health Care, 1949–69 / 109

6 'Once Upon a Time There Was No Frank Miller' / 131

APPENDIX I: Lady Superintendents and Administrators, Owen Sound General and Marine Hospital, 1893–1985 / 141

APPENDIX II: Board Presidents, Owen Sound General and Marine Hospital Trust / 142

NOTES / 143

INDEX / 157

# Illustrations

PHOTOGRAPHS
(*following page xiii*)

Dr Charles Barnhart
G&M hospital showing 1893 (left) and 1911 (right) wings
G&M hospital, 1893
Private room, circa 1914
Semi-private ward, circa 1914
Operating-room, circa 1914
Clinic, circa 1918
Tea-time, from a ward diet kitchen, circa 1920
Nurse and new arrival, circa 1920
Nurses taking a break on the roof, circa 1920
Owen Sound medical men, 1922
Hon. MacKinnon ('Mac') Phillips, MD, MPP
G&M hospital showing (l–r) 1911, 1929, and 1957 wings
G&M hospital showing (l–r) 1893, 1911, 1929, and 1957 wings
Aerial view of G&M hospital (looking west), 1963
Demolition (1963) of war surplus nurses' residence
Aerial view of G&M hospital (looking southwest), 1975

Illustrations

TABLES

1 Summary statistics, G&M Hospital, 1893–1914 / 31
2 Average length of patient stays (whole days) by diagnostic categories, G&M Hospital, 1894–1916 / 33
3 Frequency (per cent) of admissions by diagnostic classification, G&M Hospital, 1894–1916 / 35
4 Origins and sex of patients admitted, G&M Hospital, 1894–1916 / 38
5 Summary statistics, G&M Hospital, 1915–29 / 64
6 Admissions, patient stays, income, and expenditures, Ontario public general hospitals, 1880–1950 / 80
7 Comparative frequency of admissions/discharges by diagnostic categories, Ontario hospitals, 1900–47 / 83
8 Summary data, G&M Hospital, 1930–9 / 89
9 Patterns of hospital morbidity, selected disease categories, G&M Hospital, 1930–40 / 100
10 Summary data, G&M Hospital, 1940–50 / 103
11 G&M Hospital workforce, 1930–52 / 113
12 Summary data, G&M Hospital, 1949–64 / 124
13 Cases treated, G&M Hospital, 1950–63 / 127

FIGURES

1 G&M births/100 live Owen Sound births, patient fees as per cent of annual income, and surgical cases as per cent of all admissions, G&M Hospital, 1894–1929 / 39
2 Contributions (per cent) to total annual income by source, Ontario public general hospitals, 1880–1946 / 42

# Preface

This project was conceived by my friend Dr George Chamberlain who practised medicine at the Owen Sound General and Marine Hospital and who was concerned that the history of that now defunct institution might be lost to memory. The history of the G&M that follows is probably more, and less, than George bargained for. It is certainly less than he expected to the extent that it does not dwell on the customary iconography of the history of medicine as it used to be written – heroic surgeons, wise and avuncular GPs, selfless nurses, harrowing medical ordeals, scientific miracles, and assorted institutional 'characters.' It may be more than he bargained for to the extent that I have borrowed, as a model for this study, much of the recent work by historians and sociologists in the 'social history' of medicine.

This approach seeks to understand the historical relationship between those who required health care and those who provided it, not just between patients and their physicians, but, in the case of hospitals in particular, between the changing health care needs of whole communities and societies and the political, professional, institutional, and popular responses to those needs. This sort of history puts the emphasis on the relationships among social need, social policy, and social medicine. It requires the historian to try to understand the social, economic, and cultural circumstances that have periodically redefined society's assumptions about the purpose, the nature, and the results of hospital-centred medical care, the motivation behind the responses of those who provided hospital care – doctors, nurses, administrators, trustees, and benefactors – and the role of politicians in translating these periodic redefinitions of social need into formal expressions of social policy.

This may appear to be too grand a design for the history of a small town hospital. However, it is only through the histories of specific institutions such as the Owen Sound General and Marine Hospital that it is possible to see in detail the interplay of the various forces that led to the emergence of the modern public general hospital everywhere. The 'G&M' is a more or less ideal microcosm of the development of public general hospitals in Ontario after 1880, just as Owen Sound and its immediate hinterland is an ideal laboratory of changing community perceptions of, and responses to, hospital-based health care, precisely because the G&M was not the Toronto General which, because of its size, location and wealth probably was unique and atypical.

Perhaps not. The social history of medicine, and more particulary the history of the modern hospital, are not very well-developed fields of research in Canada. Only when many more such studies have been undertaken and their results synthesized will it be possible to say how 'typical' the historical development of the G&M actually was. I hope that I have succeeded in marrying my interest in the G&M as an example of the emergence of the modern hospital in Ontario with enough of George Chamberlain's interest in the G&M as an expression of something fundamentally important about the history of Owen Sound to satisfy both of us, and anyone else interested in a community's historical determination to invest its hospital with the aura of 'the single most important institution' in its midst.

In the course of completing this project I have enjoyed the support and assistance of several people, whose help I gratefully acknowledge. Garth Pierce, the president of the Grey Bruce Regional Health Centre, and his staff cheerfully allowed me to intrude on their busy routines compounded by the problems of launching a major health centre, and made the task of sorting out the G&M's records much less difficult than it might have been. Carol Vamplew, my research assistant, toiled among admissions registers and reels of microfilmed newspapers with a minimum of direction and got it all right. I am especially indebted to Izetta Fraser, whose amazing collection of historical newspaper clippings related to Owen Sound and the hospital saved me much time and effort. Betty Warrilow facilitated access to the obituaries compiled by Frances Warrilow for the Surname Collection for Grey and Bruce counties, and Stephen Meinhardt generously allowed me to share his research notes on doctors' perceptions of hospitals between 1880 and 1910. The University of Toronto Press's staff and manuscript readers helped me to avoid many pitfalls. Dr Rosemary Gagan not only helped with the research but improved the manuscript immensely with her blue pencil. Finally, I would like to thank the Board of Governors of the Grey Bruce Regional Health Centre for their support of this project.

David Gagan
11 April 1990

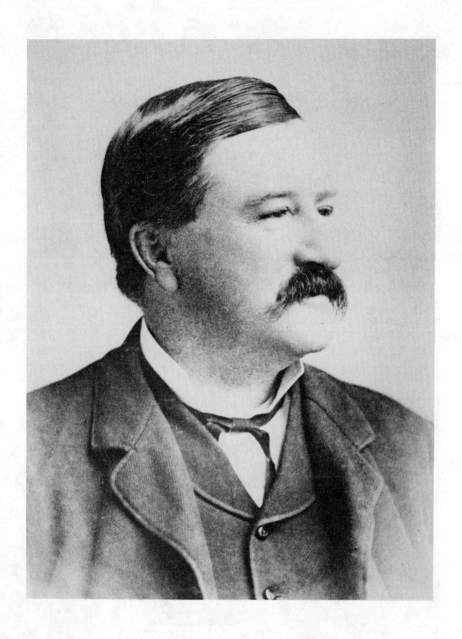

Dr Charles Barnhart (courtesy County of Grey–Owen Sound Museum)

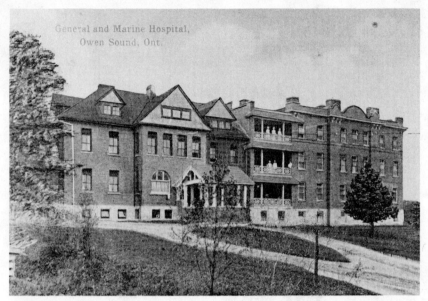

G&M hospital showing 1893 (left) and 1911 (right) wings (courtesy County of Grey–Owen Sound Museum)

G&M hospital, 1893 (courtesy County of Grey–Owen Sound Museum)

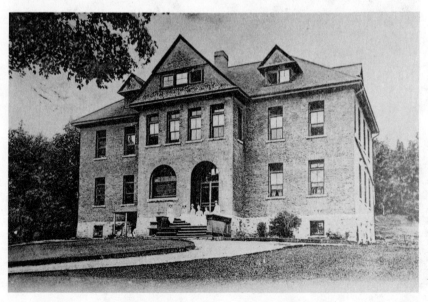

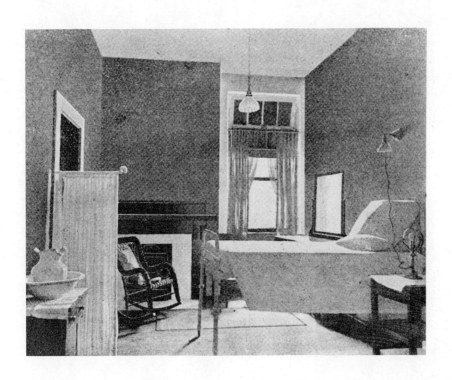

Private room, circa 1914 (courtesy Grey Bruce Regional Health Centre)

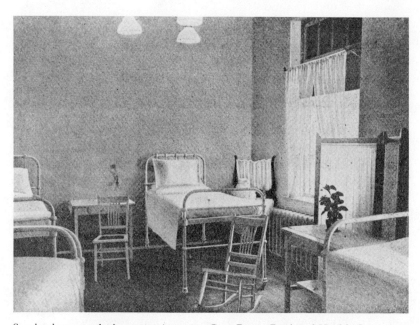
Semi-private ward, circa 1914 (courtesy Grey Bruce Regional Health Centre)

Operating-room, circa 1914 (courtesy Grey Bruce Regional Health Centre)
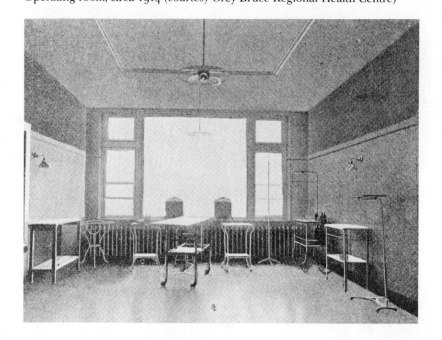

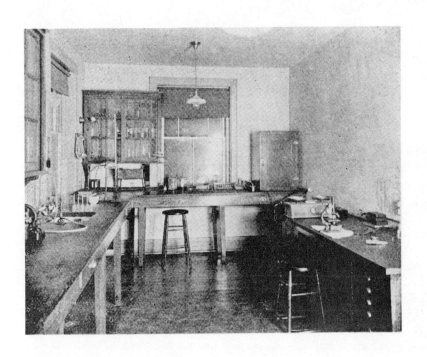

Clinic, circa 1918 (courtesy Grey Bruce Regional Health Centre)

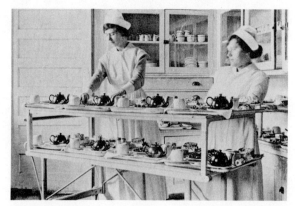

Tea-time, from a ward diet kitchen, circa 1920 (courtesy Grey Bruce Regional Health Centre)

Nurse and new arrival, circa 1920 (courtesy Grey Bruce Regional Health Centre)

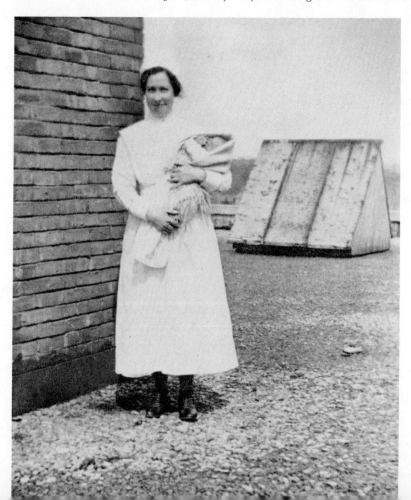

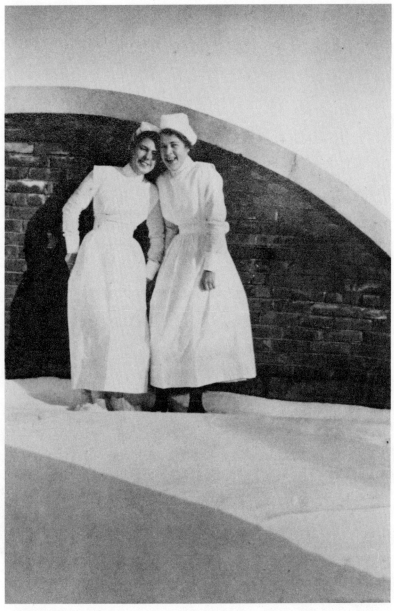

Nurses taking a break on the roof, circa 1920 (courtesy Grey Bruce Regional Health Centre)

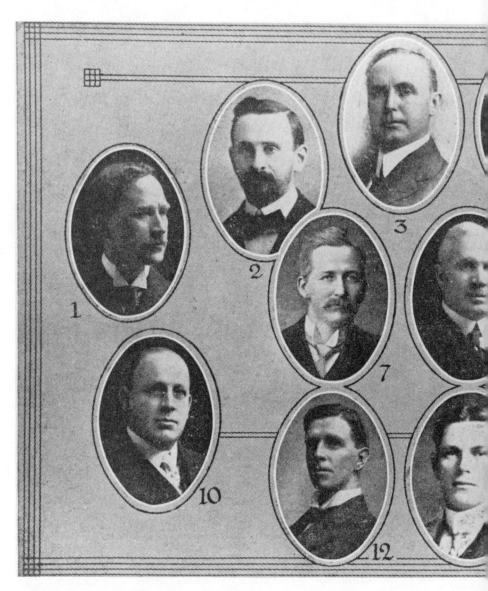

Owen Sound medical men, 1922: (1) R. Howey, (2) G.S. Burt, (3) A.L. Danard, (4) T.H. Middlebro, (5) A.B. Rutherford, (6) W.T. Frizzell, (7) W. McDonald,

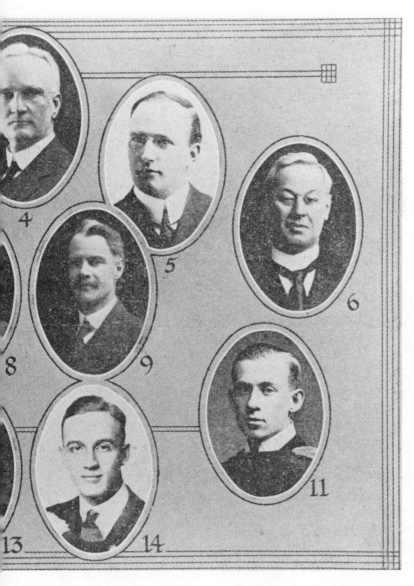

(8) W.G. Dow, (9) E.E. Evans, (10) F.A. Brewster, (11) C. Gaviller, (12) H.G. Murray, (13) G. R. Miller, (14) G.M. Fraser (courtesy Grey Bruce Regional Health Centre)

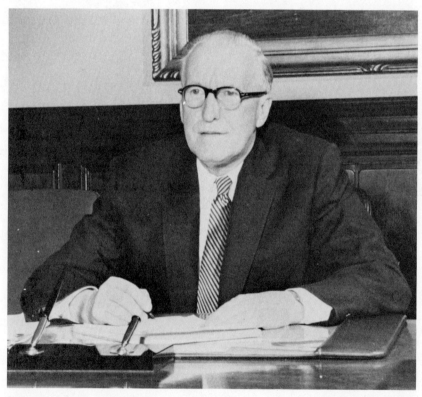
Hon. MacKinnon ('Mac') Phillips, MD, MPP (courtesy Grey Bruce Regional Health Centre)

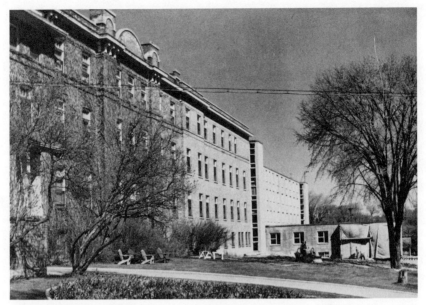

G&M hospital showing (l-r) 1911, 1929, and 1957 wings (courtesy *The Sun-Times*)

G&M hospital showing (l-r) 1893, 1911, 1929, and 1957 wings (courtesy *The Sun-Times*)

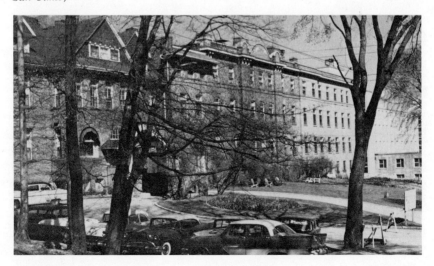

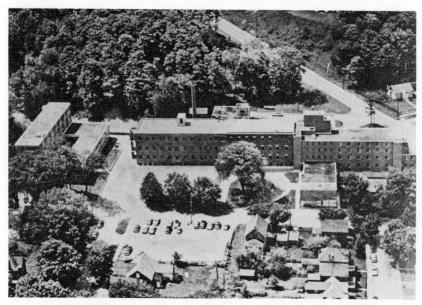

Aerial view of G&M hospital (looking west), 1963 (courtesy County of Grey–Owen Sound Museum)

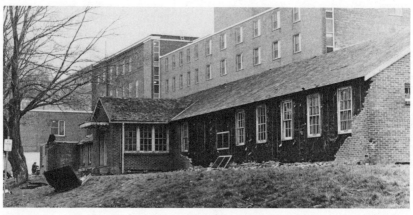

Demolition (1963) of war surplus nurses' residence (courtesy *The Sun-Times*, Owen Sound)

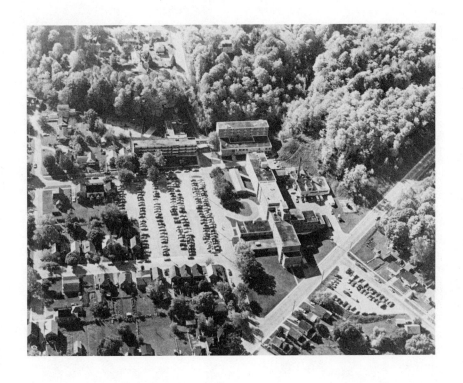

Aerial view of G&M hospital (looking southwest), 1975 (courtesy *The Sun-Times*)

'A NECESSITY AMONG US'

# 1
# 'A Great Opportunity of Doing Good': Founding the G&M, 1885–93

The town and county councils attended in a body. The president of the board officiated. The ladies' association sold souvenirs. The representatives of the butchers, the grocers, the Freemasons, the King's Daughters, the Busy Bees, and the church young people's groups who had volunteered provisions and furnishings, and the citizens, great and small, who had subscribed to the building fund, inspected the 'neat, clean and bright' wards. The mayor of the town, John Frost, reminded them all of their fundamental Christian obligation: 'To be good, it [is] necessary to do good. To be happy, it [is] necessary to make others happy. Hospitals,' he concluded, '[afford] a great opportunity of doing good.'[1] In this fashion the Owen Sound General and Marine Hospital was officially opened on the afternoon of 21 June, 1893. Six weeks later, the hospital admitted its first patient, cast up by the human tide, the 'great floating population without homes of their own,' that had become Owen Sound's reason for being and the proper object, in Mayor Frost's view, of the citizenry's charitable impulses.

Owen Sound, in 1893, was one of the twelve busiest ports on the Great Lakes, a rival, at least in terms of its water-borne commerce, of much larger ports such as Chicago and Buffalo. The source of the town's prosperity was the mobilization, in a local context, of those same forces that were responsible for three decades of eco-

4 'A Necessity Among Us'

nomic expansion and social development on a national scale after 1880. Three events, more than any others, dominate the social and economic history of late Victorian Canada. The first of these is the widespread dissemination throughout southern Ontario of urbanization and industrialization. Stimulated by the development of an efficient rail transportation network, surplus capital, and a growing market-place for domestically produced goods, the results of the province's healthy agrarian economy and by the presence of a large unskilled labour force, the growth of industrial towns from Perth in the east to Chatham and Sarnia in the west was the source of late Victorian Ontario's social and economic vitality. At the same time, an ambitious national experiment was launched with the opening of the Canadian West to settlement, first Manitoba in 1870, then the prairie wheatlands after 1885 following the construction of the Canadian Pacific Railway. To land-poor Ontario wheat farmers, to their landless sons, and to a new generation of European immigrants this vast frontier of settlement represented a Garden of Eden where free fertile land, hard work, and a bit of luck were all a man needed, it was popularly believed, to succeed beyond all hope. Finally, at the turn of the century, two great new resource frontiers, one in northern Ontario, 'New Ontario,' the other in British Columbia, yielded up their once inaccessible treasures to the incursions of the railroad. Gold, silver, copper, nickel, iron ore, timber, and enough prime agricultural land in New Ontario's Clay Belt to effectively double Ontario's inventory of arable land attracted the attention of investors, immigrants, and entrepreneurs alike.[2]

In 1893 Owen Sound sat astride these urban, western, and northern frontiers. The limestone valley of the Sydenham was a cornucopia spilling people and goods into the ship-clogged harbour that was a natural gateway to the settlements of the North Shore, to the rim of Superior and beyond to the frontier of prairie settlement an easy train ride west from the head of the lakes. Twenty years earlier, Owen Sound had been a small port town of fewer than 3500 people. Fishing, tanning, carding and flouring mills, the coastal trade, a few small foundries associated with a modest shipbuilding industry, and sawmilling augmented the town's principal economic function as the centre of commerce and services for its immediate agricultural hinterland, northern Grey and Bruce counties. The arrival of the Toronto, Grey and Bruce narrow gauge railway in 1871 was hailed as the advent of 'a new era in the history of [the] town,'[3] which now enjoyed a rail link to the south comparable to that of its nearest rival, Collingwood. With or without the railway, Owen Sound stood to benefit from the mania among southern Ontario farmers to emigrate to Manitoba in the wake of the passage of the Dominion Lands Act in 1870, and each shipping season throughout the next decade the roads leading to Owen Sound were choked with the horses and wagons of migrant Ontario farm families bound, via steam or sail, for Prince Arthur's Landing and the Dawson Road to Manitoba.[4] As the result of this stimulus, the population of Owen Sound grew by about a third between 1871 and 1881. Then, like so many other aspects of Canadian life in the first great era of national economic expansion, the town encountered the major engine of that development, the Canadian Pacific Railway Company.[5]

Shortly after its incorporation the CPR acquired a 99-year lease of the Toronto, Grey and Bruce Railway, widened the track to standard gauge, and built a major terminus in Owen Sound. Then in 1885, in fulfilment of its rights and obligations to initiate shipping services wherever its tracks terminated at a navigable body of water, but also in order to keep its own rail construction crews on the transcontinental line north of Superior supplied on a regular basis, the CPR designated Owen Sound as the home port of a fleet of five fast steamships plying a regular schedule between southern Ontario and the Lakehead.[6] The impact of this decision on the town was immediate. New industries sprang up, attracted by fast, cheap, and efficient communication not only with the North West but with major ports all around the Great Lakes, and by the town's easy access to the natural resources of the North Shore. Existing industries expanded. Owen Sound became a major centre for forwarding, grainhandling, fish gathering, victualling, sawmilling, and furniture manufacturing and, by 1895, was the principal Canadian source of Portland cement, boasting three major plants around its harbour and, 30 miles to the south, the largest marl cement-manufacturing plant in North America. In 1888 a Toronto shipbuilder opened in Owen Sound the first shipyard on the Upper Lakes to build iron steamships; to man it he brought from Scotland the Clydeside shipbuilders who had built the first three CPR steamers to sail out of Owen Sound. Georgian Bay, La Salle's Mer Douce, was the town's life blood for the next 25 years. Between 1881 and 1893 the population of Owen Sound nearly doubled in response to this outburst of new opportunities. But the size of the town's rapidly growing permanent population paled in comparison to the much larger population of sailors, migrants, teamsters, tourists, drummers, entertainers, navvies, and lumbermen for whom Owen Sound, which by 1891 had begun to style itself as the 'Liverpool of Canada,' was simply a traveller's way station. Numbers are difficult to estimate, but, for example, in the year between 1 July 1888 and 30 June 1889, 1171 vessels passed in and out of Owen Sound harbour. Their crews alone consisted of about 24,000 men.[8] In addition, the CPR steamers, not to mention their smaller rivals, could transport a total of nearly 2000 passengers a week on their outward voyages.

It was this 'floating population' of thousands of sojourners from every walk of life that gave the town its atmosphere of exuberant vitality and some of its less desirable characteristics. In 1890 there were 13 licensed drinking establishments in Owen Sound, one for every 130 adult males; but at least one unlicensed hotel sold whisky by the pailful out the back door after hours. The *Times* complained in December 1888 that an epidemic of drinking and poker-playing would lead the youths of Owen Sound to ruin, and the editor welcomed the end of the navigation season as instant relief from 'wandering drunks' and 'prowlers.'[9] But if the seasonal flow of transients (and some of their less appealing diversions), the frenzy of activity in the harbour, and the booming commercial prosperity of Poulett Street gave Owen Sound the aura of a raw frontier town, it was also a community intent on becoming modern in the best sense of the Victorian idea of progress.

The measure of progress was the material and moral condition of the people, and the improvement of both was the subject of widespread public debate in Victorian Ontario. Much of that debate focused on the need to reconcile the apparent contradiction between the material benefits that accrued to communities from the activities of unrestricted free enterprise and the prevailing Christian gospel that material progress without social responsibility was unethical.¹⁰ In Toronto, municipal elections in the 1880s and 1890s were decided, more often than not, by the relative persuasiveness of one side of that argument or the other.¹¹ Among smaller towns like Owen Sound and its rivals – Stratford, Guelph, Brantford, Galt, and Berlin – whose 'boosters' worried that failing to keep abreast of civic developments and attitudes elsewhere would compromise their town's attractiveness to industrialists and merchants, the need to marry the interests of private and public good was no less compelling. 'Public improvement is an investment that pays,' the editor of the *Times* admonished his fellow citizens in the autumn of 1888. 'Get at it.'¹²

In 1893 there was much to admire about civic development in Owen Sound. The Collegiate Institute, established in 1880 as a teacher-training facility, was reputedly one of the best high schools in the province, and there were two lending libraries containing nearly 6000 frequently borrowed volumes. The spires of at least two recently built, handsome churches, Knox Presbyterian and St George's Anglican, dominated the prospect of the town from Frost's Hill, and the county court house and gaol, the town hall with its cupolaed clock tower, and a first-class hotel – the Paterson House – offered solid bricks-and-mortar evidence of the town's architectural maturity. A home-building boom in the mid-eighties expanded the town's stock of fine residences and promoted an aura of middle-class pride in permanence. In 1890 the streets of Owen Sound were lit by hydroelectricity generated by the Owen Sound Electric Illumination and Manufacturing Company's plant at Inglis Falls, six miles south of the town. Ten years earlier the company's partners had successfully built Owen Sound's water system, tapping natural springs in the limestone formations surrounding the town. The arrival of not one but two telephone companies in 1884 and the completion of the Grand Trunk's spur line from Park Head in 1893 rounded out Owen Sound's full complement of public and private utilities.¹³

The city's material development was matched by its citizens' interest and involvement in the major social questions of the day. In the same year, 1874, that the Woman's Christian Temperance Union was launched in Cleveland, its first Canadian branch was organized in Owen Sound.¹⁴ Similarly, in 1893 Owen Sound, as the county seat of Grey County, was one of the first communities in Ontario to respond to the call of the great child-saver, J.J. Kelso, to create a children's aid society for the prevention of cruelty to children. Its local mentor, the Reverend James Lediard, became one of the foremost social reformers in Ontario.¹⁵ A city of churches with a strong bent towards church-centred social activism, Owen Sound provided the first two permanent missionaries to West China sponsored by the Woman's Missionary Society of the Methodist Church of Canada.¹⁶ As for the widespread debate between the supporters of unrestricted free enterprise and the proponents of a society in which competition was tempered by a spirit of social and economic co-operation, Owen Sound and Grey County were the focus of much of the activity of the Dominion Grange movement in the 1880s. A nationwide fraternal society of farmers organized to promote, especially through farmers co-operatives, a higher standard of living for farmers and a united agrarian lobby in matters of national policy, the Grange benefited from the leadership of men like R.J. Doyle, a pioneer cement manufacturer who edited and published *The Canadian Co-operator and Patron* from 1881 until 1903. Doyle also managed the Dominion Grange Mutual Insurance Company, headquartered in Owen Sound, on behalf of Canadian farmers, and his wife was the moving spirit behind the local WCTU.¹⁷

These developments were consistent with Owen Sound's ambition to present itself as a progressive community. The state of the town's public health was not. Judging by the nature and extent of newspaper commentary on the subject, public health in Owen Sound was neither better nor worse than in any other urban centre in late Victorian Ontario; but that says a great deal about it. By 1885 concern about the health threat to Ontarians from epidemic diseases had become so widespread that the government created a provincial board of health. Its mandate was to collect statistics, to educate the public, and to superintend the work of local boards of health and their medical health officers in their struggle against disease and its breeding grounds, unclean water, contaminated food, inadequate sanitation, bad housing, overcrowding, poor personal hygiene, and industrial pollution.[18] Smallpox, tuberculosis, diphtheria, typhoid fever, and infant mortality were particular targets of a public health system that, given the state of public and scientific ignorance, could only respond to immediate crises without much hope of permanent successes.[19]

In Owen Sound, threats to citizens' health and, therefore, to their social well-being seemed to arise from several recognizable causes which were more apparent to the editor of the *Times* than to the local medical health officer, Dr Allan Cameron. The first of these was the city's failure to regulate the producers and vendors of food and milk. Butcher shops and dairies were the worst culprits because they sold their products directly to unprotected consumers who then suffered the consequences, including death, of eating contaminated meat and drinking impure milk. But the condition of the slaughterhouses on the west side of the harbour was no less scandalous. They sluiced their offal directly into the bay. The situation in the town's residential districts was no better. Householders were permitted to run sink drains directly into roadside gutters, and there was no system for collecting household garbage. Since the city refused to enforce its cow by-law (there were nearly 900 cattle and 232 hogs within the town limits in 1890), cattle roamed and grazed at will, adding to the noxious wastes that accumulated from a horse-intensive transportation system serviced by several livery stables, whose sanitation methods were also unregulated. For the hundreds of migrants who passed through town on their way west, there was near the CPR station a single public well and trough which served every purpose. It had to be closed temporarily in 1888 when it was used to wash the clothing of a typhoid victim; the medical health officer suspected that it was used regularly for unsanitary purposes in any case, although he could do nothing about the problem.[20]

The *Times* thought that the medical health officer was too passive and that the board of health, which rarely met, was indifferent to conditions in the town. It was certainly true that in 1890 the death rate in Owen Sound was nearly twice the rate for rural Grey County, and that perhaps as many as 45 per cent of those deaths were attributable to causes associated with public health problems. As he later explained, Dr Cameron was indeed circumspect about his part-time duties as medical health officer because the office was incompatible with his need to maintain a private practice in order to earn a living. Patients preferred doctors who were not exposed on a daily basis to the epidemic diseases feared by the whole community.[21] Of these, the almost annual autumn visitation of typhoid fever gave the townspeople the greatest cause for concern. It was not until 1927 that the city's water supply was identified as the carrier, and chemical treatment of the water put an end to the annual epidemics. In the meantime, Cameron and his successors struggled each year to contain the spread of typhoid and other dreaded diseases, such as diphtheria, smallpox and scarlatina through the usual practice of isolating active cases. It was this strategy that led to the first proposal to establish a permanent hospital in Owen Sound, an isolation hospital, in response to a particularly severe epidemic of typhoid in 1885, when a vacant house was rented for quarantine purposes.[22]

When the idea next surfaced, in 1889, it had become a project of the town's physicians and was no longer envisaged as merely an isolation hospital, but rather as a voluntary public general hospital where philanthropic medical treatment could be provided to the sick poor and people of limited means according to their ability to pay. There is very little documentation that might help to explain why Owen Sound's physicians collectively took up the cause of a voluntary public general hospital or how they managed to enlist the aid, then the leadership, of some of the town's wealthiest and most influential citizens in this enterprise. What seems certain is that, quite apart from the problem of infectious disease, Owen Sound's 10 active physicians found it increasingly burdensome, as the town's permanent and transient populations grew, to cope in their surgeries with the escalating numbers of acute treatment cases, especially those arising from industrial, shipping, and railroad accidents, all the more so if the patients happened to be strangers in the town who could not be cared for subsequently in a private home. Some were sent to the Toronto General Hospital, while others were undoubtedly entrusted to the care of the two private nurses who resided in the town.[23] Whatever the case, when the physicians' representatives appeared before the town council in January 1889 to promote their scheme, they took pains to assure the aldermen that their motive was strictly philanthropic and not prompted by professional self-interest. At the ninth hour, when it appeared that the scheme might fall apart, the argument used to rally popular support for it was that, without the hospital, Owen Sound would fall behind its rivals in its communal commitment to public charitable work.[24]

All of these motives – the isolation of contagion, the care of strangers, charitable care for the sick poor, the institutionalization of the community's spirit of voluntarism, and, ultimately, the identification of the hospital as the most appropriate physician's workshop in certain cases of illness – were common elements in Victorian society's gradually changing perception of the role of the hospital. Hospitals were a phenomenon of the urbanization and industrialization of western society at the end of the eighteenth century. Particularly as they developed in England, the United States, and Canada, hospitals existed to provide medical charity, usually in the form of simple custodial care, to the sick poor. No respectable person who could afford private medical care would willingly set foot in a hospital, if only out of fear of contracting an illness – pyemia or erysipelas for example – more life-threatening than the reason for admission. But in fact the middle classes neither required nor sought admission because income, family structure, the availability of domestic servants and private nursing, and their physical environment made home care safer than institutional treatment. However, for the urban poor in times of sickness, neither short-term nor chronic care was possible in overcrowded households organized only for work. It was for this increasingly visible element of the population that the voluntary general hospital became a widespread urban institution in the nineteenth century.

Some of these public general hospitals were municipal institutions funded and managed by city councils. Others were sponsored by religious orders. Most were the creatures of voluntary committees of public-spirited citizens. Financed through public and private subscriptions and donations, voluntary hospitals were administered by boards of governors elected or appointed from among their wealthiest patrons. Subscribers controlled admissions through their right to nominate deserving patients, who in turn required the patronage of a subscriber to gain admission. Once admitted, the sick poor were literally in the custody of an institution which either killed them or from which they emerged no better than when they had entered. Hospital infection was rampant. Nursing care, until Florence Nightingale's reforms of the 1870s, was in the hands of ignorant and illiterate domestic servants whose ministrations were more to be feared than admired. Physicians, who served voluntarily, were generally unable to intervene in any purposeful way to improve the patient's condition. The essential purpose of hospital administration, usually the responsibility of a matron, was to enforce rigidly the rules governing the behaviour of patients, to keep characteristically unruly staff in order, and to hoard the hospital's usually inadequate supplies. For much of the nineteenth century the hospital was a fundamentally Dickensian institution in which the well-being of needy patients was almost incidental to its reason for existence as defined by its patrons, lay administrators, medical consultants, and paid functionaries.[25]

In the late Victorian era, however, the hospital came under the influence of profound forces of change. The first of these was the revolution in the quality of hospital care introduced by Florence Nightingale and her disciples, for whom efficient hospital and patient management at the hands of trained nursing professionals was measured in terms of the patient's physical well-being and the quality of the environment in which healing took place. The second was the revolution produced by Listerism, that is, the introduction of antiseptic and aseptic procedures which drastically reduced the risk of hospital infections and made the hospital a less threatening environment for the patient. But the most important consequence of this discovery was an era of surgical advancements which, perhaps more than any other factor, transformed the hospital into a necessary adjunct of the physician's art. Together with vastly improved diagnostic techniques, for example as the result of the introduction of x-ray technology at the turn of the century, successful surgical intervention in cases of acute suffering produced both the need and the justification for a suitable new environment in which the teaching and the practice of 'scientific' medicine could take place. Coincidentally, towards the end of the nineteenth century the urban middle classes began to discover the modernizing hospital as an acceptable alternative to increasingly problematical home care, even as their private physicians were hotly debating whether hospital privileges were essential to successful medical practice. Consumer demand, professional elitism, and the obvious therapeutic benefits of hospital-centred medical science conspired to redefine the hospital as a 'workplace for the production of health'[26] for all members of the community. This implied new priorities for admitting patients to hospital including, as medical technology became more expensive, the ability to pay for treatment. By the turn of the century, private and semi-private rooms for paying middle-class patients had begun to be incorporated into hospitals everywhere.[27] Health care was becoming a marketable commodity. Hospitals, once charitable institutions, now the necessary 'embodiments of modern medical science,'[28] helped to create the growing market economy in health care where none had existed before.[29]

Voluntary associations nevertheless remained the commonest form of hospital organization in England, the United States, and Ontario. This was partly because the tradition of voluntary communal support of a non-denominational, non-political, non-profit and still charitable institution maintained primarily for the sick poor continued to play an important role in the middle class's perception of the hospital as a testament to their Christian and civic duties. As well, in the absence of any state-supported schemes of medical care, fees collected from those patients who could afford to defray some or all of the rapidly rising costs of institutionalized health care were inadequate to support the hospitals' charitable responsibilities. Voluntary fund-raising was therefore still an essential aspect of hospital economics. But increasingly, voluntary boards of trustees were confronted by the preoccupations of the new breed of professional managers that hospitals required, by the medical profession's changing perception of the proper role of hospitals in society and of doctors in hospitals, and perhaps above all by patients' changing expectations of the quality and objectives of hospitalization.[30] Once the hospital ceased to be associated with the stigma of pauperism, the aura of the charnel house, and the futility of treatment and became the preferred source of acute medical care for all classes of the population, it also came under intense public scrutiny as the place where the modern family divested itself of the responsibility for dealing with problems of life and death.[31] Voluntary stewardship then became synonymous with the obligation to underwrite the costs of a cultural revolution directed by forces essentially beyond the control of the civic-minded volunteer.

This transition was just beginning to take shape when the idea of a public general hospital was first discussed in Owen Sound. In 1890, for example, there were only 20 public general hospitals in Ontario concentrated in 15 communities. The total number of patients admitted represented less than one per cent of the population of Ontario.[32] Fewer than 500 births took place in these institutions in 1890, and only 600 deaths occurred. The nearly 10,000 patients admitted spent on average more than 30 days in hospital but less than 20 per cent of their maintenance was charged directly to them. In fact, 90 per cent of the days of care required by these patients was subsidized by the provincial and municipal governments under the Charity Aid Act (1874) which provided for annual provincial grants-in-aid to hospitals of 20 cents per day for all patients and 25 cents for indigent patients.[33] All of this suggests that even in 1890 hospital care in Ontario was largely the preserve of the poor and the indigent who were admitted for essentially custodial care. Although it was a teaching hospital and therefore not wholly typical of its lesser counterparts in smaller places, the largest hospital in the province, the Toronto General, was financed almost exclusively by private donations and government grants, and admitted inpatients only on a nomination basis from its founding in 1829 until 1881. Medical privileges were restricted to the General's staff of appointed voluntary attending physicians and surgeons drawn largely from the University of Toronto's medical faculty. It was not until 1881 that the hospital finally gave in to the demands of private physicians that they be allowed to admit their private paying patients to the hospital, to attend to them personally there, and to collect fees for doing so,[34] in effect ending the General's role as a primarily charitable institution.

This scenario was replayed at different times in different places, partly depending on local priorities, but more generally as the result of the gathering momentum among Canadian physicians between 1890 and 1910 to restrict the practice of medicine to highly qualified graduates of recognized medical schools, to create a clientele willing to pay for 'scientific' medical treatment at the hands of these skilled practitioners, and to provide those physicians with professional advantages denied to the 'irregular' practitioner and his patients. In this struggle for professional hegemony, the hospital increasingly was identified as a critically important asset in the inventory of scientific medicine. For example, in the 1870s the *Canadian Lancet* – the principal organ of the medical profession in Canada – characterized hospitals as repositories of disease for the instruction of medical students and the relief of the poor, but otherwise unfit for general use, for surgery, or for patients who could afford private care.[35] Thirty years later, the journal's commentators were arguing that the hospital was a place where physicians, even in small towns, could acquire the broadest possible clinical experience, a place where the public (as both visitors and patients) could be educated in the principles of modern health care, a place where the pooled resources of many doctors working together, learning from and supporting each other, produced better care, where the scientific practice of medicine did not discriminate among its beneficiaries, and, not least of all, a facility in which all physicians had an equal right to treat their private paying patients as well as an equal obligation to dispense medical charity to the poor.[36] By the turn of the century, then, both the medical profession and consumers of medical science had a vested interest in the redefinition of the scope and objectives of hospital-based medical care, but it is safe to assert that everywhere in Canada vestiges of the Victorian hospital, including the stigma of poverty attached to hospital admission, persisted well into the first two decades of the twentieth century.

This was the milieu that undoubtedly shaped and influenced private and public perceptions of the role and character of a hospital for Owen Sound when the local medical men enlisted the support of the town council and several of the town's leading citizens in 1889. The moving spirits were Dr Allan Cameron, the medical health officer for Owen Sound; his counterpart in Sarawak Township, Dr Charles Barnhart; Dr James McCullough who practised in the village of Chatsworth nine miles south of the town; and Dr George Dow, formerly house surgeon and resident *accoucheur* at the Toronto General. By early February 1889 they had succeeded in developing a concrete plan for a hospital and attracting a grant of $1000 from the Grey County Council, payable after the building was completed.[37] After a special committee had considered the matter for two weeks, the Owen Sound Town Council pledged $600 from its revenues, another $1000 from a bequest left in trust to the town for charitable purposes, and a parcel of land in the south end of the town.[38] With these pledges in hand, the committee, Dr Cameron later reminisced, attracted the attention of Stephen J. Parker, Frederick d'Orr Le Pan, and William Roy, who joined them in creating a hospital trust to receive voluntary donations. Parker was the entrepreneur behind the town's water system and the Electric Illumination and Manufacturing Company. Eventually he also created the town's gas distribution system. Le Pan, Parker's father-in-law, moved to Owen Sound from Illinois in 1847 and became the owner of the town's largest hardware store. William Roy was reputedly the richest man in Owen Sound. Born in Dumfrieshire, Scotland, he emigrated to Montreal, made a fortune in commerce, and at the age of 47 'retired' to Sarawak Township, although he found time to create the Royal Loan and Savings Company of Brantford and the Owen Sound and Grey and Bruce Loan and Savings Company of which he was president. S.J. Parker was vice-president.[39]

By 1891 Roy, Le Pan, Cameron, and Parker with two of their closest associates, John Harrison, proprietor of the largest sawmill in Owen Sound, and J.M. Kilbourn, a barrister and private banker, had become the moving forces behind the hospital scheme which, after two years of voluntary fund-raising, seemed close to becoming a reality. The decision was taken in the spring to incorporate the hospital trust, solicit tenders for the construction, and possibly even begin to build during the summer. Slightly more than $6000 had been pledged, and of that a little less than $3500 had been received.[40] But the committee (later the board of trustees) had failed to reckon with the opinions of their subscribers and the sensitivities of their most energetic fund-raisers, the Ladies' Hospital Aid. Twice the Ladies' Hospital Aid arranged joint meetings with the men's committee to draw up the terms of incorporation of the hospital trust and twice the men failed to appear, having, in fact, privately drawn up an instrument of incorporation which excluded women from voting membership in the trust and, therefore, from the board of trustees. The *Times* reported on 6 July 1891 that the ladies were 'desperate' and were considering withdrawing their support from all fund-raising activity. This action would have dealt a serious blow to whatever momentum the project had gathered as a public enterprise, because it was the ladies' program of continuing events – teas, concerts, recitals, charity balls and socials – that kept the idea of a hospital in the public's mind as a communal project rather than as the private philanthropy of a few of the town's leading citizens. The women's anger must have had domestic repercussions as well, insofar as the most active members of the ladies' association were the wives and elder daughters of the physicians, merchants, industrialists, and bankers most closely identified with the hospital project. Eventually the Ladies' Aid was partially mollified by a public vote of thanks and, more significantly, by an (apparently) informal agreement that representatives of the Ladies' Aid would be seconded to the House Committee of the hospital, giving them, in effect, a voice in the daily management of the institution. The impasse was resolved temporarily, but within six months of the official opening of the hospital, the Ladies' Aid had become so dispirited that its executive considered resigning *en masse* and finally decided to withdraw from all direct involvement in the management of the hospital.[41]

The subscribers to the trust, many of whom had not honoured their pledges when the board of trustees met formally for the first time in May 1891, were less tractable. The board had hoped to call for tenders even before a site had been confirmed, but at a subscribers' meeting held on 3 June the board was instructed to resolve the site issue first. The difficulty was that the town council had offered free land in the industrialized south end of town while board members expressed individual preferences for either the 'Pleasure Grounds' on the east hill above the town or the old 'market square' on Bay Street just east of the harbour. Subscribers preferred the more central Bay Street location, and the board petitioned town council to seek a patent for the land, which was still vested in the

Crown. The summer passed with no response from the commissioner of crown lands. Finally, in frustration the board's site committee recommended the purchase of a large park lot a considerable distance north of the town's centre on the west side of the harbour. It is not clear why the Brownlee property, for which the board paid $3000 in the form of a mortgage at 6 per cent for 10 years, was considered preferable to the free land offered by the town. One explanation is that a site close to the community's 'great floating population' was deemed essential. It also provided ample room for future expansion and, in the meantime, for an essential garden, an orchard, and pasturage for the hospital cow. The site also ensured that fever patients would not be housed close to the town's preferred residential areas. The subscribers finally approved the site and authorized its purchase, and on 8 September 1891, the board directed Allan Cameron and a local architect to visit hospitals in Guelph, Stratford, Brantford, and Galt in order to ascertain the best features of modern hospital construction. Meanwhile the board set to work drafting by-laws and adopting the official seal of the corporation with its motto, 'Heal the Sick.'[42]

The board decided to adapt the plan of the Galt Hospital to suit the available resources and called for tenders in late September. To their chagrin the bids submitted 'far exceed[ed] the expectations of the subscribers,' who had hoped to erect their hospital for about $8000. The lowest bid, $8127, included neither plumbing nor heating. With unpaid pledges of $4000, cash on hand totalling $1500, and the promise of $2500 in grants and legacies as its only working capital, the board had no choice but to scale down its plans in order to bring the total project in under $8000. The plans were revised, and the board received bids of $5494 from a local contractor, Alex Greene, for the building, and $1703 for plumbing and heating from Christie and Agee. The contracts were signed on 12 March 1892, and building commenced when fine weather returned in the spring.[43]

In its final form the hospital was a two-storey brick structure built, in the words of the provincial inspector of charities, in a 'good plain and substantial style,' with an attic, a full basement, hot-water heating, and gas lighting in the wards. The kitchen, laundry, and storerooms were in the basement; nurses and servants were housed in the attic. Each of the two main floors contained both public and private wards. The operating room was on the second floor; the superintendent's office and private rooms, as well as the common dining-room, were on the main level. The inspector took particular note, during his visit on 13 February 1893, of the plumbing, which was 'of the most modern description. Bath rooms and water closets are provided on each flat. The water supply is from the town system.' During a subsequent visit on 18 August the inspector, Dr F. Chamberlain, noted that the hospital required a morgue, a dispensary, and a disinfecting room, all of which could be housed in a shed at the rear of the building. These minor problems aside, the 'well-managed Hospital' with its 'good staff of medical officers and nurses' was recommended for inclusion by order-in-council in Schedule A of the Charity Aid Act. This made the hospital eligible to receive a perpetual provincial subsidy of up to 30 cents per day for each non-paying patient treated and, for its first 10 years of operation, a similar subsidy for all paying public ward patients to a maximum of 25 per cent of the hospital's total annual revenue.[44] Between the inspector's two visits, that is, between the completion of construction and the admission of the Owen Sound General and Marine Hospital's first patient, there was more than enough cause for anxiety among its supporters. In spite of a vigorous last minute fund-raising campaign by the indefatigable Ladies' Hospital Aid, by mid-May the board faced a serious financial crisis. Unpaid pledges meant that the contractors' accounts could not be settled. Nor could the board provide salary advances for the hospital's newly appointed caretaker and his wife, who was to serve as both cook and laundress. A 'most discouragingly attended' subscribers' meeting, called to rally flagging enthusiasm for the project, fell apart when a quorum of trustees failed to attend, convincing the *Times* that the hospital might never open. Two weeks later the corporation's annual meeting drew an equally disappointing turn-out, prompting the new president, S.J. Parker, to comment that not even the town's doctors who had been 'the instigators of the scheme' seemed interested any longer in their creation. In fact, the medical men had to be invited to meet privately with the board to discuss staffing arrangements for the hospital; it was the middle of June before they 'signified their intention of assisting in the benevolent work and routine of hospital duty,' finally volunteering to establish week-long duty shifts in return for being enrolled as the hospital's staff governed by regulations of their own devising. No sooner had the doctors been brought on side than the caretaker and cook tendered their resignations, apparently because they still had not been paid. Moreover, it was the end of June before the board was able to recruit a suitable lady superintendent, Miss J.E. Moore, to manage its increasingly tenuous enterprise.[45] In the meantime, the G&M had been officially opened on 25 June to the strains of Holland's Orchestra playing optimistic music while subscribers in arrears quaffed refreshments.

When at last the hospital admitted its first patient in mid-August, five months behind schedule, new obstacles arose to test the resolve of the board. Almost immediately a member of the medical staff lodged a formal complaint against Miss Moore, accusing her of being disrespectful to a patient who had objected to being served mouldy bread. The dispute was less trivial than its immediate cause might suggest. The administrative structure of the Owen Sound General and Marine Hospital, as laid down in the hospital's *Rules and Regulations*, was a relatively simple one common enough among Victorian hospitals. Responsibility for the day-to-day management of the hospital was vested in the lady superintendent. She ordered all supplies, provisions, and medicines, kept an account book for each of the hospital's commercial suppliers and another for donations in kind, hired and fired nurses and domestic staff, superintended the quality of nursing and domestic care, and regulated the social behaviour of patients. Except for the necessity of providing the secretary of the board with a monthly statement of her accounts, reporting nursing misconduct to the board and the visiting physician, and seeking the approval of the visiting physician before removing a patient for wilful misconduct, the lady superintendent exercised virtually unrestricted authority over her domain.[46] In the mid-nineteenth century, this concentration of authority in the hands of a single paid administrator had served the purposes of an institution operated as a voluntary medical charity interested primarily in the social control of indigent patients. But as hospitals increasingly became identified, especially in the minds of physicians, with active medical intervention to heal the sick, an inevitable conflict arose between the prerogatives of doctors and the managerial responsibilities of lady superintendents who, by the end of the century, represented the emerging new profession of hospital administration. Just as inevitably, boards of voluntary lay trustees found themselves caught in the middle.[47]

A special committee of the board struck to investigate Dr Brown's complaint reported in October that Miss Moore had never acted in an intentionally disrespectful manner toward either patient or physician, as had been claimed. Pleading for 'harmony and good feeling among all those who are united together for the common purpose of making this charity an unmixed benefit to the Town and community,' the committee recommended 'a little forbearance and mutual respect' among staff members.[48] It was not to be. A month later the board received a second complaint, from a seriously ill nurse who was supported by Dr Dow, that Miss Moore had refused to permit a private physician to attend the nurse and, moreover, had prevented the nurse's friends – the other nurses employed at the hospital – from visiting her (she had a fever of 104 degrees Fahrenheit and was probably contagious). Matron Moore insisted that she was carrying out the wishes of the nurse in question and her responsibilities as the nurse's supervisor. Dr Dow demanded a written apology from both Miss Moore and the board for allowing his and his patient's rights to be abrogated.[49]

The board of trustees reluctantly concluded that Miss Moore had not adhered strictly to regulations. Citing ill health, overwork and 'the fact that the Assistance given me is entirely inadequate,' on 24 November Miss Moore submitted her resignation and departed for Toronto as soon as her bags were packed, leaving the hospital, patients, and staff unsupervised. Four days later a letter from Dr Chamberlain, the inspector of charities, arrived advising the board that it would be necessary for him to investigate certain problems arising from Miss Moore's resignation, problems which might lead to the decertification of the hospital. The inspector arrived on 2 December, claiming no acquaintance with Miss Moore but some knowledge of her fine family background and a more detailed familiarity with the unsanitary condition of the hospital and the incompetence of the nurses responsible for it. He departed the next day, having given explicit instructions that a morgue, a laundry, an incinerator, and a sanitary sewer line to carry the hospital's 'simply harmless' effluent directly to the bay must be constructed immediately if the board wished to retain the hospital's accreditation.[50]

It was an expensive lesson in the politics of Ontario's developing social services bureaucracy and an illustration of the transitional state of hospital and medical professionalism. Chamberlain represented the provincial inspector of prisons and public charities, a title which reflected traditional Victorian perceptions of the character and objectives of hospitals in society. But as its annual reports suggest, the inspectorate was remarkably forward-looking in the 1880s and 1890s. For example, it actively discouraged the foundation of municipally operated civic general hospitals on the grounds that the sick, especially the sick poor, should not be the pawns of municipal politics and politicians. Consequently inspectors promoted voluntary associations of public-spirited citizens as the best way to ensure a 'high degree of excellence' in hospital care[51] – one of the reasons, undoubtedly, why the voluntary public general hospital became the commonest form of hospital organization in Ontario. Similarly, inspectors were not sympathetic to the idea that physicians should manage or interfere in the administration of hospitals and were clearly aware and supportive of the revolution in administrative and nursing professionalism wrought by Florence Nightingale and her disciples in the very recent past. 'There are now available in this country,' one inspector noted as early as 1885, 'ladies of ability and experience, who have been systematically trained in nursing and the domestic management of hospitals, any of whom would be abundantly capable of taking full charge of the whole internal economy of [an] Institution ... and manag[ing] it better [than a Medical Superintendent].'[52] Nevertheless, there were dangers to be apprehended when professional nurses invaded the physician's domain. As one inspector explained, 'training schools for nurses are affecting a great revolution in hospital management ... [S]till it is not unknown ... to find nurses who are trained just a little too much. It is a somewhat hazardous thing to engraft upon an imperfectly trained intellect too much technical knowledge ... There is a danger of training out the woman and the nurse, and leaving behind a mischievous female doctor.'[53] Victorian gender biases dictated that insofar as the domestic economies of hospitals, overseen by 'boards of ... gentlemen,'[54] were simply the domestic economy of the family household writ large, their management and the care of their patients represented woman's proper and natural sphere. A scientific knowledge of medicine was not. These biases notwithstanding, Dr Chamberlain and his fellow inspectors were interested in the efficient, economical, and professional management of hospitals and patients in receipt of provincial funding. Skilled professionals, in the office of the lady superintendent, were their obvious preference as administrators, whose cause Chamberlain and his colleagues were ever ready to champion.

Ironically, in the wake of this setback the board of the General and Marine Hospital turned to the only woman doctor in Owen Sound, Eliza Gray, who temporarily took charge of the hospital while the board sought applications from prospective matrons. At last it appointed Miss R.E. McKenzie, supervisor of the Toronto General's Gynecological Pavilion (which was larger than the G&M), a nurse recommended by her superintendent and the General's resident surgeon as 'uniformly conscientious and capable and possessed of good executive ability.'[55] Matron McKenzie lived up to her advanced billing; with the assistance of three nurses, a domestic servant, a part-time laundress, a cook, and a porter, by the spring of 1894 she had the hospital 'in that first-class condition which its promoters always hoped it should occupy.' From the board's point of view, 'the crucial period [had] been passed, the prospects for the future [were] bright.'[56]

The hospital that the citizens of Owen Sound had thus created was a voluntary public general hospital conceived as a charitable institution for the care of the sick and homeless poor. Provision was made for the admission, in the usual Victorian fashion, of indigent and other patients suitable for free treatment. Indigent patients required a signed certificate of admission from the elected head (reeve, mayor, warden) of any municipality eligible, through its financial support of the hospital, to nominate patients for admission. But any person could be nominated for free treatment by the president of the board of trustees, or by any individual, society, or business which had contributed sufficient funds to the trust to qualify for the right to nominate patients. In 1893 a donation of $100 entitled the contributor to nominate patients for the equivalent of one patient-year of treatment. The exceptions were chronically ill patients and maternity cases. The former would not knowingly be admitted to the hospital, and the latter could not be admitted unless they had resided in Owen Sound for at least six months prior to parturition, and then only for a maximum of two weeks of care. In this way, the hospital evidently hoped to discourage long-stay non-paying patients who tied up beds needed for acute care. The hospital's rules thus reflected the changing perception of the role of hospitals in relation to the emerging medical profession's developing ability to intervene effectively in the treatment of acute illnesses. The G&M's rules for admission gave clear precedence to accident victims, patients requiring surgical treatment, and patients with treatable acute diseases.

The regulations governing admissions also anticipated the admission of paying private and semi-private ward patients under the care of their personal physicians if the doctor held a staff appointment in the hospital. Together with the provision, in the construction of the hospital, for a small number of private and semi-private rooms, these regulations suggest that at least some middle-class patients and their physicians were already accustomed to the idea of hospital care as a viable, and in some cases preferable, alternative to home care. But it is equally possible that the trustees had simply anticipated a preference for special care, including 'expensive wines, medicines and fruit,' by the better class of travellers heading west and in need of medical attention.

One reason for drawing this conclusion is that the regulations governing the medical staff required them to treat free of charge any patient who was content with the services of the physician on duty. In effect, only the standard of accommodation, not the quality of medical care, was predicated on the ability to pay. Moreover, once a doctor had undertaken the care of a patient as part of his week-long duty shift, he continued, with the agreement of the patient, to be the attending physician until the patient was discharged. In this way patients of all classes were guaranteed not only free but consistent treatment within the expanding limits of current medical knowledge and practice, which was also regulated in the interests of patients' welfare. From the outset the medical staff of the G&M imposed limitations on their colleagues' freedom to treat patients, requiring prior consultation with a majority of the staff in all cases of proposed surgery, and the concurrence of a majority of those consulted on the diagnosis and the surgical intervention recommended.

Patients admitted for treatment found themselves confronted by the 'discipline of the hospital' which evidently had less to do with creating a therapeutic environment than with the apprehension of social disorder and inculcating an ethic of institutional efficiency and social utility. Free patients were admitted under a general injunction to show the necessary respect at all times to the officers, employees, and medical staff of the hospital, and to obey the orders of the lady superintendent, the nurses, and the medical officer on duty. Loitering, dancing, whistling, card playing, profanity, chewing or smoking tobacco, quarrelling with other patients, wearing a hat, and resting fully clothed on a hospital bed were all forbidden activities. Drinking spirituous liquor was sufficient cause for immediate discharge. Patients were required to remain in bed between the hours of 9:00 PM and 6:30 AM. During daylight hours ambulatory indigent patients were expected to undertake any work, for example cleaning the wards, assigned to them by the lady superintendent. Free patients could have visitors Tuesdays, Fridays, and Sundays, and ministerial visitors at any time. No patient was constrained, however, to participate in any religious observances or activities except on a voluntary basis. None of these rules seems to have applied to paying patients, who were even permitted to have overnight guests; it would be many years before a preponderance of paying patients, and changing social perceptions, mitigated the compulsion to assign a higher priority to the social than to the medical regulation of patients' activities.[57]

This enterprise was the responsibility of the Owen Sound

General and Marine Hospital Trust, a publicly incorporated charity of which any citizen could be a life or annual member upon nomination and the payment, respectively, of either a $100 or $2 fee. Members of the trust elected annually 13 of their number who, with the mayor of Owen Sound and the warden of Grey County's delegate, constituted the board of trustees who elected from their own number the officers of the trust and formed its standing committees. The Building and Grounds Committee was responsible for the physical plant, the House Committee for the daily operations of the hospital.[58] Within this context, much of the board's routine work fell on the shoulders of its secretary-treasurer (the first was John Tolton, an accountant), who was in daily contact with the lady superintendent and with her constituted a very effective, if informal, management committee. The remaining members of the board were not, however, merely corporate window dressing. In an earlier age they might have been content to wear their voluntary stewardship lightly as a natural consequence of their patronage of the sick poor; but as the process of establishing a public general hospital unfolded, so did the perception that this was not simply an asylum for the sick poor, but an investment in the standard of living of the whole community. To succeed it required more than perfunctory instalments of noblesse oblige. It required active participation in the work of funding, promoting, managing, improving, and defending the investment as the most important secular charity in the county. It therefore required the ministrations of volunteers undeterred by the gulf that separated popular perceptions of the hospital's historical identity from the vision of what it might become.

The Owen Sound General and Marine Hospital had not been conceived by its founders on the model of the emerging modern hospital that had moved 'from treating the poor for the sake of charity to treating the rich for the sake of revenue.'[59] But neither was it a classically Victorian 'instrument for grudging and inexpensive relief of the sick poor, an agency of social control, and an arena for the professional aspirations of elite physicians.'[60] The G&M occupied the middle ground shared by its sister institutions in the nascent Canadian system of voluntary general hospitals. They offered preferential care to the small minority of their patients who could pay for it in order to provide, with the assistance of individual, municipal, and provincial generosity, a minimum standard of care to the vast majority of their clients who required hospitalization in spite of their inability to pay, and because of personal circumstances that made private care impossible. But even as this system of voluntary general hospitals was rapidly taking form and direction from these impulses between 1890 and 1914, it was already beginning to encounter new forces of technological, economic, and cultural change which would fundamentally redefine the mandate, the clientele, and the economics of the community hospital.

In 1893 it was enough that the people of Owen Sound and northern Grey County had come to the realization that a general hospital, as a response to rapid urbanization, as an agency of social improvement, as a desirable object of private and public charity, and as a symbol of civic pride, had simply become 'a necessity among us.'[61]

# 2
# 'A Public Utility': The Emergence of the Modern Hospital, 1893–1914

The history of the Owen Sound General and Marine Hospital's first quarter-century is a microcosm of the transformation of general hospitals throughout North America, between 1890 and 1930, from marginally useful agencies of medical charity into socially and medically indispensable centres for the scientific treatment of disease. This transformation was brought about, after 1890, by the interplay of many forces. Medical science and technology made rapid advances in the diagnosis and treatment of disease, especially the development of safer and more effective surgical techniques for which the hospital was the only suitable venue. Coincidentally, domestic life was undergoing fundamental changes. The modern family became less willing and able to accept responsibility for the care of convalescents, and the family soon proved less capable of caregiving than the new profession of nursing. Especially for those who could afford the preferential care which hospitals increasingly offered, either as an inducement to or in response to the expectations of a paying clientele, the benefits of hospital treatment were powerful stimulants to the development of a popular perception of the hospital as the primary health care centre. At the same time, the movement on the part of physicians to be recognized as an exclusive profession characterized by the practice of scientific medicine also promoted the hospital as the medical professional's essential workshop where his private patients would reap the benefits of treatment by teams of skilled specialists with recourse to better equipment, facilities, and support services than the individual physician could provide in his office.

The result was not merely a transformation, but a revolution in hospital admissions, standards of care, costs, sources of income, and public relations which took place in a remarkably short period of time, perhaps no more than 30 years. The consequences of that revolution, however, had to be worked out over a much longer term and are still unfolding. Almost from the outset, voluntary boards of hospital trustees were faced with the same problems governments face today: accessibility, funding, and cost effectiveness in relation to the quality of medical care. By 1914 all of these factors had come into play in Ontario's emerging health care system, no less so in the Owen Sound General and Marine Hospital than in any of its larger metropolitan sister institutions.

In the beginning, the G&M was conceived and operated on the model of the Victorian hospital, a response to the social problems of rapid urbanization. It was an isolation facility during periods of epidemic disease attributable to the town's unhealthy environment. It was an emergency treatment facility necessitated by the growing number of shipping and, especially, railway accidents as the volume of traffic through the port increased dramatically. It was a refuge for sick sojourners for whom domestic care was impossible. It was even a temporary asylum for town drunks and lunatics. But above all the Owen Sound General and Marine Hospital was first conceived, built, and promoted as a place where individual and familial poverty and sickness, 'a combination too strong to be fought single-handed,' could become the collective responsibility of the whole community and its superior resources – fiscal, medical, and moral. The hospital, no less than the home, the school, and the church, was to be 'an influence for good on the lives of all who enter [its] gates.'[1]

Within 10 years these priorities had given way to the perception of the G&M as first and foremost a 'centre for the treatment of disease,' especially through surgical intervention, among all classes of the population.[2] Its effectiveness was already being measured in terms of patient demand, income, administrative efficiency, and its ability to provide the latest innovations in medical technology and convalescent care. A decade later, certainly by the end of the First World War, the G&M's transition from medical charity to medical workshop was virtually complete. It had become, according to its own publicity, the best hotel in the county patronized by the best citizens in the community, who recognized that it was 'no reflection on home' to prefer the quality of treatment and care provided by 'the most useful and necessary [institution] in the town.'[3]

The most obvious gauges with which to measure the progress of this transition are the patterns of patient usage which were both the cause and the effect of the general hospitals' changing image. The number of patients admitted to the G&M (see Table 1) increased at an average annual rate of about 20 per cent during the hospital's first decade of operation, but this growth was not exponential. In both 1896–7 and 1902–3, for example, admissions dropped below previous levels as the result, in both instances, of the unpredictable course of public health in the community. The late summer months of 1897 were virtually free of epidemic disease and the hospital was underutilized relative to its customary overcrowding during the town's recurrent epidemics. On the other hand, a particularly severe outbreak of typhoid (46 cases) in 1902 produced a glut of long-stay patients which limited the total number of patients who might have been admitted during the year.[4] Even as late as 1916 a double-edged epidemic of typhoid and scarlet fever filled the G&M's medical wards to overflowing and severely restricted the hospital's more recently acquired preference for surgical and obstetric cases. These events underscore the extent to which the G&M's original functions as a custodial and convalescent facility continued to define and sometimes restrict its role in the community even as the hospital was becoming a centre for the treatment of acute disease. From this perspective, the years between 1904 and 1908 seem especially critical. Both the number of patients seeking admission and the reasons for their admission suggest that the G&M was beginning a new stage in its growth and development. The hospital was seen by both patients and staff to be constantly overcrowded. Moreover, this increased activity, which soon had strained the hospital's resources to the limit, was clearly associated, in the minds of the medical staff, the nursing staff, and the board, with two new phenomena: an

TABLE 1
Summary statistics, G&M Hospital, 1893–1914

| | Year ending 30 September | | | | | | | | | | |
|---|---|---|---|---|---|---|---|---|---|---|---|
| | 1894 | 1896 | 1898 | 1900 | 1902 | 1904 | 1906 | 1908 | 1910 | 1912 | 1914 |
| No. of patients treated* | 66 | 112 | 133 | 213 | 263 | 290 | 360 | 305 | 377 | 436 | 546 |
| Total patient days | 1,899 | 3,280 | 4,560 | 4,768 | 6,466 | 7,503 | 7,119 | 5,504 | 7,256 | 6,999 | 6,973 |
| Average stay | 28.8 | 29.3 | 34.3 | 22.2 | 24.6 | 25.9 | 19.8 | 18.0 | 19.2 | 16.1 | 16.6 |
| Total operating income ($) | 2,286.40 | 2,229.08 | 3,158.78 | 5,507.79 | 3,671.31 | 6,730.13 | 6,255.39 | 7,440.03 | 9,142.59 | 14,567.57 | 13,507.68 |
| Municipal grants ($) | 91.66 | 345.39 | 850.00 | 930.00 | 1,225.00 | 1,285.00 | 824.85 | 1,825.00 | 2,275.00 | 2,175.00 | 3,205.35 |
| % of income | 4.0 | 15.5 | 26.9 | 17.2 | 21.6 | 19.1 | 13.2 | 24.5 | 24.9 | 14.9 | 23.7 |
| Provincial grants ($) | 550.15 | 767.75 | 986.8 | 803.72 | 1,019.50 | 826.78 | 645.82 | 666.74 | 830.31 | 743.42 | 636.27 |
| % of income | 24.1 | 34.4 | 31.2 | 14.6 | 18.0 | 12.3 | 10.3 | 9.0 | 9.1 | 5.1 | 4.9 |
| Subscriptions ($) | 988.78 | 348.84 | 409.37 | 2,351.06 | 855.57 | 1,586.08 | 967.68 | 1,245.51 | 479.59 | 4,622.55 | 490.23 |
| % of income | 43.2 | 15.6 | 13.0 | 42.7 | 15.1 | 23.6 | 15.5 | 16.7 | 5.2 | 31.7 | 3.6 |
| Patient fees ($) | 655.81 | 767.10 | 912.61 | 1,403.01 | 2,571.24 | 3,032.27 | 3,817.04 | 3,702.78 | 5,557.69 | 7,026.60 | 9,155.83 |
| % of income | 28.7 | 34.4 | 28.9 | 25.5 | 45.3 | 45.1 | 61.0 | 49.8 | 60.8 | 48.2 | 67.8 |
| Total operating costs ($) | 1,766.51 | 2,264.56 | 2,898.37 | 2,975.58 | 4,272.16 | 6,796.60 | 5,648.57 | 7,401.15 | 8,065.06 | 13,598.01 | 11,731.34 |
| Cost of food ($) | 550.26 | 637.65 | 719.60 | 714.34 | 1,286.62 | 1,681.59 | 1,415.38 | 1,862.32 | 2,392.00 | 4,416.33 | 4,010.44 |
| % of costs | 31.1 | 28.2 | 24.8 | 24.0 | 30.1 | 24.7 | 25.1 | 25.2 | 29.7 | 32.5 | 34.2 |
| Supplies and services ($) | 1,216.25 | 1,626.91 | 2,178.77 | 2,261.24 | 2,985.54 | 5,115.01 | 4,233.19 | 5,538.83 | 5,673.06 | 9,181.68 | 9,117.46 |
| % of costs | 68.9 | 71.8 | 75.2 | 76.0 | 69.9 | 75.3 | 74.9 | 74.8 | 70.3 | 67.5 | 77.7 |
| Patient fees as % of operating costs | 37.1 | 33.3 | 31.5 | 47.2 | 60.2 | 44.6 | 67.6 | 50.0 | 68.9 | 51.7 | 78.0 |
| Income per patient day ($) | 1.20 | 0.68 | 0.69 | 1.16 | 0.88 | 0.90 | 0.88 | 1.35 | 1.26 | 2.08 | 1.94 |
| Cost per patient day ($) | 0.93 | 0.69 | 0.64 | 0.62 | 0.66 | 0.91 | 0.79 | 1.34 | 1.11 | 1.94 | 1.68 |
| Usage (% of capacity) | 12.1 | 20.9 | 29.1 | 30.4 | 41.2 | 47.8 | 40.6 | 31.4 | 41.4 | 32.0 | 31.8 |
| No. of surgical cases | 20 | 21 | 21 | | | | 100 | 150 | 137 | 182 | 187 |

*Excludes newborns
SOURCES: Sessional Papers of Ontario; Annual Reports, G&M Hospital

upsurge in the number of paying patients demanding better accommodation and treatment facilities than the hospital could offer, and a significant increase in the number of surgical cases.[5] It was to accommodate both of these developments that the hospital was expanded in 1911. Although large increases in user fees (necessitated by rising costs), the pre-war recession, the war itself, and, as in the past, seasons of good public health all contributed to significant annual variations in admissions, the number of patients treated nearly quadrupled between 1910 and 1919.

Annual admissions, however, can be misleading indicators of the hospital's level of activity, tied as they are to the hospital's constantly fluctuating capacity in relation to the number of beds actually available for active treatment and to the length of time each patient occupies a bed. Thus, one reason for the steady increase in admissions, quite apart from (but no doubt partly responsible for) the growing acceptability of hospitalization, was the coincidental decline in the average duration of patient stays from more than 30 days in 1893 to about two weeks in 1916 (see Table 2). In the absence of effective therapeutic treatment, either through surgery or with drugs, the hospital's first patients commonly stayed until their disease had run its course or until hospitalization was no longer useful and they were sent home to die. Similarly, the preponderance of indigent and homeless patients among the hospital's earliest clientele promoted prolonged stays while the patient convalesced. In time, more rapid convalescence was facilitated by less traumatic surgical techniques, better nursing care, and changing perceptions of the treatment of convalescent patients. Table 2 suggests that the hospital developed particular efficiency in the management of maternity patients, surgical cases (those classed under genito-urinary, digestive, and to a lesser extent nervous and sensory system), and certain respiratory disorders. But the G&M also became more rigorous in its exclusion of chronically ill patients as time passed. No doubt paying patients' reluctance to subsidize unnecessarily prolonged hospital stays in the face of rising charges also contributed to the more rapid turnover of patients and beds. Whatever the cause, the result was to reduce dramatically the average length of a stay and, theoretically at least, almost to double

TABLE 2
Average length of patient stays (whole days) by diagnostic classification, G&M Hospital, 1894–1916

| Diagnostic category | Hospital year ending on 30 September | | | | | | | |
|---|---|---|---|---|---|---|---|---|
| | 1895 | 1898 | 1901 | 1904 | 1907 | 1910 | 1913 | 1916 |
| All patients | 30 | 30 | 26 | 25 | 20 | 19 | 19 | 16 |
| Infective & parasitic | 29 | 30 | 30 | 18 | 21 | 23 | 15 | 21 |
| Neoplasms | 28 | 18 | 16 | 21 | 16 | 14 | 15 | 18 |
| Allergic, endocrine, etc. | n/a | 49 | n/a | 19 | 36 | 13 | 25 | 23 |
| Diseases of blood & blood-forming organs | 2 | 6 | n/a | 35 | 13 | n/a | 18 | n/a |
| Mental, psychoneurotic | 6 | 46 | 21 | 19 | 18 | 9 | 23 | 11 |
| Diseases of nervous system & sensory organs | 30 | 49 | 11 | 30 | 13 | 18 | 20 | 21 |
| Diseases of circulatory system | 57 | 37 | 22 | 11 | 20 | 13 | 17 | 13 |
| Diseases of respiratory system | 32 | 28 | 36 | 12 | 16 | 11 | 8 | 14 |
| Diseases of digestive system | 19 | 27 | 24 | 26 | 19 | 20 | 18 | 18 |
| Diseases of genito-urinary system | 34 | 24 | 18 | 14 | 12 | 20 | 19 | 21 |
| Delivery, complications of pregnancy, puerperium | 22 | 27 | 16 | 21 | 17 | 14 | 14 | 12 |
| Diseases of skin & cellular tissue | 32 | 36 | n/a | 12 | 32 | 49 | 14 | 16 |
| Diseases of bones & organs of movement | 38 | 23 | 38 | 25 | 20 | 21 | 34 | 32 |
| Congenital malformations | n/a | n/a | n/a | n/a | 14 | n/a | 22 | 3 |
| Certain diseases of early infancy | n/a | n/a | n/a | 4 | n/a | n/a | n/a | 7 |
| Symptoms, senility | n/a | n/a | n/a | 121 | 365 | 20 | 16 | 27 |
| Special admissions | n/a | 44 | 27 | 26 | 15 | 46 | 28 | 2 |
| Accidents/poisonings/violence | 30 | 12 | 27 | 33 | 35 | 31 | 15 | 27 |
| Not stated | 21 | 31 | 32 | 55 | 18 | 11 | 78 | 11 |
| Live births | n/a | n/a | 14 | 12 | 23 | 11 | 12 | 12 |

between 1893 and 1905 the number of patients the hospital could treat annually without physically expanding its facilities.

The usual measure of actual hospital capacity and use is the patient day. If one patient day is defined as one patient occupying one bed for one day, then the actual annual capacity of the G&M in patient days prior to 1911 was 15,695 (43 beds × 365 days) and subsequently 21,900 (60 × 365), excluding newborn infants. Between the opening of the hospital in 1893 and its first major expansion in 1911, hospital usage, measured in patient days, increased from 12 per cent to nearly 50 per cent of capacity (Table 1). It would appear at first glance that the hospital was never more than half full. In practical terms, however, a 50 per cent level of utilization meant that during its busiest seasons – fall, winter, and in particular during the annual typhoid or scarlatina epidemics – the hospital was overcrowded and there were waiting-lists of patients. By 1905 these lists tended increasingly to consist of patients awaiting not only surgery but the availability of private or semi-private accommodation; hence the need both to increase the hospital's capacity, in spite of the added capacity created by reductions in hospital stays, and to upgrade its accommodations and treatment facilities to reflect the needs of a changing clientele.[6] Ironically, expansion, the vastly increased fees required to finance it, and the continuing reduction in patient stays combined to create a brief but painful admissions crisis on the eve of the First World War. In fact it was not until the end of the war that hospital usage once again approached anything like 50 per cent of capacity. Even so, there were still, from time to time, serious strains on the hospital's space as the focus of the G&M's burden of work shifted even more rapidly than before from its now underutilized medical ward to its busy surgical and obstetrics wards.

Table 3 presents the timing and the extent of this fundamental redefinition of the hospital's character in terms of changing patterns of hospital morbidity.[7] Unfortunately, no patient discharge records survive for the G&M, so hospital morbidity must be inferred from the reasons given for admission and from incomplete annual summaries of diseases treated. Even so, the extent to which the G&M primarily fulfilled during the 1890s its original purpose as a fever hospital is unmistakable. Less obvious from the aggregated data are the number of admissions during the 1890s representing complications arising from tuberculosis, and beds occupied by chronically ill (usually destitute elderly) patients, many of them awaiting admission to the county home. Early in the new century these patterns began to change. In particular, the increasingly accurate diagnosis of and successful surgical treatment for diseases of the digestive tract, which produced the first great modern era of antiseptic surgery, were largely responsible for redefining the role of the General and Marine Hospital. This process began, coinciden-

TABLE 3
Frequency (per cent) of admissions by diagnostic classification, G&M Hospital, 1894–1916

| Diagnostic category | Hospital year ending on 30 September | | | | | | | |
|---|---|---|---|---|---|---|---|---|
| | 1895 | 1898 | 1901 | 1904 | 1907 | 1910 | 1913 | 1916 |
| No. of patients admitted | 83 | 135 | 262 | 315 | 335 | 401 | 469 | 555 |
| Infective & parasitic | 22.9 | 25.9 | 29.8 | 18.7 | 14.0 | 17.7 | 8.7 | 9.4 |
| Neoplasms | 6.0 | 5.2 | 3.1 | 3.2 | 5.4 | 4.0 | 4.3 | 2.0 |
| Allergic, endocrine, etc. | 0.0 | 0.7 | 0.0 | 0.6 | 0.9 | 1.0 | 2.1 | 1.4 |
| Diseases of blood & blood-forming organs | 1.2 | 0.7 | 0.0 | 0.6 | 1.2 | 0.0 | 0.9 | 0.0 |
| Mental, psychoneurotic | 4.0 | 5.2 | 6.5 | 8.9 | 2.4 | 4.5 | 2.3 | 2.5 |
| Diseases of nervous system & sensory organs | 7.2 | 5.9 | 0.8 | 4.1 | 6.0 | 6.7 | 4.5 | 4.9 |
| Diseases of circulatory system | 7.3 | 5.9 | 3.5 | 3.8 | 3.9 | 2.5 | 3.4 | 1.3 |
| Diseases of respiratory system | 10.8 | 6.7 | 8.8 | 10.2 | 10.4 | 9.2 | 4.9 | 12.3 |
| Diseases of digestive system | 3.6 | 5.9 | 17.2 | 9.8 | 16.7 | 16.7 | 22.4 | 16.6 |
| Diseases of genito-urinary system | 7.2 | 7.4 | 9.5 | 5.4 | 11.9 | 7.7 | 12.2 | 4.1 |
| Delivery, complications of pregnancy, puerperium | 4.0 | 4.4 | 3.1 | 6.3 | 5.1 | 7.7 | 10.7 | 13.5 |
| Diseases of skin & cellular tissue | 6.0 | 6.7 | 0.0 | 4.8 | 2.4 | 1.0 | 0.4 | 1.6 |
| Diseases of bones & organs of movement | 7.2 | 6.7 | 4.2 | 4.8 | 3.1 | 4.0 | 3.4 | 1.6 |
| Congenital malformations | 0.0 | 0.7 | 0.0 | 0.0 | 1.5 | 0.0 | 0.4 | 0.2 |
| Certain diseases of early infancy | 0.0 | 0.0 | 0.0 | 0.6 | 0.0 | 0.0 | 0.0 | 0.5 |
| Symptoms, senility | 0.0 | 0.0 | 0.0 | 3.2 | 0.6 | 0.5 | 0.6 | 0.7 |
| Special admissions | 0.0 | 2.2 | 4.2 | 2.2 | 3.3 | 1.7 | 0.6 | 0.2 |
| Accidents/poisonings/violence | 9.6 | 7.4 | 6.5 | 7.6 | 7.8 | 7.7 | 6.8 | 6.1 |
| Not stated | 1.2 | 2.2 | 2.3 | 3.5 | 0.9 | 1.0 | 3.4 | 11.4 |
| Live births | 0.0 | 0.0 | 0.8 | 1.6 | 2.4 | 6.2 | 7.9 | 9.7 |
| No. of surgical cases | | | | 150 | 137 | | 263 | 276 |
| No. of deaths (excluding stillbirths) | 7 | 8 | 12 | 17 | 29 | 25 | 22 | 55 |
| No. of births (including stillbirths) | 1 | 2 | 3 | 8 | 8 | 25 | 36 | 68 |

tally, about the time that Drs T.H. Middlebro, W.T. Frizzell, and Richard Howey took working sabbaticals: Frizzell and Howey in London, England (to become licentiates of the Royal College of Surgeons), Middlebro in Germany, to study the latest surgical techniques which had already revolutionized the treatment of appendicitis, hernias, gall bladders, goitres, and certain gynecological disorders.[8] After 1906 surgical cases usually accounted for more than 50 per cent of all annual admissions. As the medical staff expanded and its range of surgical procedures became more diversified, and as the hospital's surgical facilities were gradually improved, abdominal, gynecological, and otolaryngological operations became the hospital's stock-in-trade with appendectomies, herniotomies, adenoidectomies, hemorrhoidectomies, and D&Cs the most common procedures.

A less dramatic, but equally important contribution to the redefinition of the G&M's mandate can be attributed to the gradually changing preference among some women and their physicians for hospital maternity care. It was not until 1927 that a majority of the births in Owen Sound occurred in hospital; it may be that the G&M's sometimes unsatisfactory record of infant mortality was itself a deterrent to expectant mothers, who preferred to give birth in the private, familiar, and comforting surroundings of their own homes.[9] But increasingly the town's physicians tended to refer especially complicated pregnancies and deliveries to the hospital, where the chances of mother and infant surviving were, arguably, enhanced. For example, the risks inherent in caesarian sections were considerably reduced in a hospital environment.[10] What is important is that the arguments on behalf of incorporating a maternity ward into the G&M were first put forward not by the medical staff but by the women of Owen Sound in 1904 through the hospital's recently re-created Ladies' Auxiliary.[11] An obstetrical ward finally was provided in the hospital's new wing in 1911. But as an adjunct of the medical ward it failed to meet the standards of privacy for mothers or to provide a separate nursery for infants, as defined by the government's rapidly changing expectations of publicly supported hospitals and by the preferences of middle-class patients as interpreted by the Ladies' Auxiliary, who maintained a proprietary interest in all matters connected with the progress of obstetrical care in the G&M. By the time these innovations were completed in 1916,[12] mothers and their newborn infants comprised nearly 25 per cent of the hospital's annual population (see Table 3). Together, obstetrics and surgery constituted the main business of the hospital by the eve of the First World War.

Among the hospital's patients, residents of Owen Sound comprised the largest single group, as might be expected. But from the outset the General and Marine was also a county hospital drawing between one-fifth and one-third of its patients from the rural townships of Grey County, especially those closest to the town: Derby, Keppel, Sarawak, Sullivan, and Sydenham (see Table 4). Distance and poor roads made it difficult for residents of the more southerly and easterly townships of the county to use the hospital. This complicated the board of trustees' annual task of securing grants from the county and township councils on the strength of the argument that the G&M was a truly regional hospital. To underscore their sincerity, between 1911 and 1916 the board of trustees briefly renamed the hospital the Owen Sound and Grey County General and Marine Hospital.[13] But to all intents and purposes it remained, from 1893 until 1939, the hospital for the area embraced by the Sydenham River's watershed, with a permanent population of perhaps 25,000. The G&M also fulfilled its founders' intention of creating a haven for the town's 'floating population' of sojourners. Especially during the first decade of the twentieth century (that is, until the CPR withdrew its fleet to Port McNicol in 1912), transients accounted for about 15 per cent, on average, of the hospital's annual patient load (see Table 4). They tended to be young single men, many of them the victims of railway, shipping, and industrial accidents.

Until 1910 the majority of patients admitted to the G&M were male. The balance shifted towards a preponderance of female patients only after the introduction of the obstetrical ward in 1911. Before and after this event, women patients, excluding obstetric cases, typically outnumbered men in only a handful of diagnostic categories – neoplasms, genito-urinary, psychoneurotic, skin and cellular diseases, and basal metabolic disorders. One reason for this pattern may be that certain gender-specific diseases, breast cancer and ovarian or uterine disorders, for example, were easily diagnosed and consequently were among the first disorders most commonly subject to surgical intervention in the early part of this century.[14] It seems, moreover, that even the women of small-town Ontario could not escape the prevalent late Victorian medical and cultural biases that prescribed unspecified periods of hospitalization for a variety of female 'complaints,' ranging from hysteria to

TABLE 4
Origin and sex of patients admitted to G&M Hospital, 1894–1916 (percentages)

| | Hospital year ending on 30 September | | | | | | | |
|---|---|---|---|---|---|---|---|---|
| | 1895 | 1898 | 1901 | 1904 | 1907 | 1910 | 1913 | 1916 |
| Owen Sound | 57.8 | 68.1 | 51.7 | 54.0 | 48.7 | 60.6 | | 61.1 |
| Grey County | 38.6 | 19.3 | 26.2 | 32.1 | 36.1 | 28.2 | | 26.1 |
| Bruce County | | | | 0.6 | 0.3 | | | |
| Other Ontario | 2.4 | 11.9 | 20.2 | 13.0 | 14.6 | 9.5 | | 5.9 |
| Other Canada | | | | 0.3 | | 0.7 | | |
| Foreign | | | 1.1 | | | | | 0.5 |
| Not stated | 1.2 | 0.7 | 0.8 | | 0.3 | 1.0 | | 6.3 |
| Male* | 61.7 | 59.7 | 57.9 | 58.8 | 52.6 | 63.8 | 48.0 | 46.6 |
| Female* | 38.3 | 40.3 | 42.1 | 41.2 | 47.4 | 36.2 | 52.0 | 53.4 |

*Excludes newborns

melancholy. Among male patients, the only equivalent causes for hospitalization were delirium tremens and senile debility. On the basis of the evidence provided by admissions records it would seem that, except for their changing attitudes towards childbirth (see Figure 1), the women of Grey County generally were less likely than men to consult a physician or, if they did, were less likely to be referred to the hospital or to accept hospitalization except for a rather limited range of disorders.

One further important characteristic of the General and Marine's admissions during this transitional era is the shift from a predominantly dependent to a largely paying clientele. At its inception the hospital presented itself as, and was seen to be, a charitable enterprise in both senses of the phrase. It received charitable donations of cash, goods, and services to fund its operations, and it dispensed charity, in the form of free or partially subsidized medical care, to anyone unable to pay the full cost of its services. In the beginning the hospital had only very limited facilities for the preferential care of paying patients in private or semi-private wards and the public wards were unlikely to attract the interest of anyone assured of domestic care. The public wards offered undifferentiated and unembellished basic care to indigents and to those paying patients who could afford the weekly maintenance charge of three dollars.

The Emergence of the Modern Hospital 39

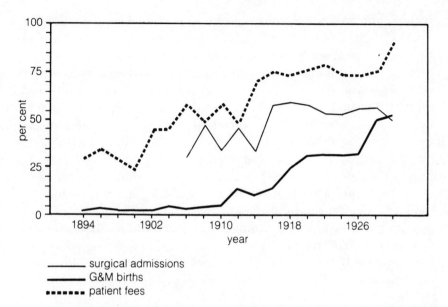

Figure 1. G&M births/100 live Owen Sound births, patient fees as per cent of annual income, and surgical cases as per cent of all admissions, G&M Hospital, 1894-1929

In a typically busy month at the turn of the century, public ward patients outnumbered private and semi-private patients four-to-one, and less than 25 per cent of the hospital's total income was derived from the fees of paying patients of any sort. Donations and government subsidies for both indigent and paying public ward patients constituted the bulk of the hospital's operating and capital funds (see Table 1). Five years later, this situation had been substantially altered. Fees paid by patients for their maintenance accounted for more than half of hospital revenues beginning in 1905 (nearly 70 per cent by 1915). In 1907 the G&M introduced the first of the historical surcharges, in this case for surgical operations performed in the hospital, which were to become permanent, and increasingly vexatious, additions to public hospitals' schedules of fees for paying patients for the next half-century.[15] Thus, in a very short time the G&M had come to depend, for its financial survival, on paying patients referred to it by private physicians (see Figure 1). But the G&M's original mandate as a charitable institution remained, and the care of indigents continued to be a major expense. The hospital's income for indigent patients, however, was determined, in the case of provincial subsidies, by statute, and in the case of municipal grants by annual agreements between the hospital and local authorities. Almost invariably these combined subsidies accounted for no more than the hospital's average per diem costs of maintaining charity cases and made no contribution to the hospital's other overheads. The year ending 30 September 1909 provides a good example of the problem. In that year, the G&M accommodated 74 indigents who represented 25 per cent of the year's admissions and 30 per cent (2094) of total patient days. (Interestingly, their average stay, 30 days, was nearly twice as long as that of paying patients.) The combined provincial and municipal grants represented income on their behalf of $1.34 per patient day, just five cents more than the hospital's average operating costs per patient day. Inevitably, fees charged to the hospital's paying clientele and income from other sources had to be adequate, if not to subsidize directly the care of indigents, then to provide the services that all patients required irrespective of their ability to pay. The necessary corollary of this development was either increased charitable donations on the part of the public or the accommodation of more paying patients in more attractive surroundings, which would justify premium rates that would produce substantially higher annual revenues. Not surprisingly, most of the new wing completed in 1911 was devoted to semi-private and private accommodation for the hospital's expanding clientele of patients willing and able to pay for differentiated, that is, preferential, care. Between 1893 and 1910 the G&M ceased to be a one-class institution as patients from all walks of life increasingly looked to institutionalized care as the source of their medical well-being. In turn, the ability not only to pay for that service but to afford user fees significantly inflated by the expectation of preferential treatment, expectations which the hospital could no longer afford to ignore, introduced class distinctions into the distribution of the hospital's resources.

Within this context of the changing role of the hospital in the community, the institutional structures, administrative policies, funding mechanisms, and planning priorities of the General and Marine Hospital were constantly reshaped to meet the needs of the community and to respond to the evolving state of medical science and technology. From the beginning, the board of trustees was necessarily preoccupied with the hospital's fiscal requirements. Meeting the institution's monthly operating expenses, discharging its mortgaged debt (a first mortgage of $3000 representing the purchase of the Brownlee site, a second of $4000 for the balance of construction costs, and another $1000 for start-up expenses), maintaining the physical plant, making desirable, or at least necessary, improvements, and providing for some capital accumulation as a hedge against unforeseen circumstances represented a tall enough order for a normal business. For an enterprise initially dependent on voluntary individual donations and subscriptions, municipal grants, and statutorily limited government subsidies for the largest share of its revenues (see Table 1 and Figure 2), fund-raising was an art just slightly more critical than cost control.

The hospital's first decade of operations consequently was characterized by an incessant campaign to involve the whole community in the process of making the G&M a financially viable operation. As Table 1 indicates, under normal circumstances the trust could expect to raise between $400 and $1000 annually through cash donations and subscriptions. Special appeals to counteract recurrent fiscal crises usually attracted the necessary public generosity. But in good times and bad the board had to be inventive in order to sustain subscriptions and donations. One strategy was to introduce several variations of the hospital by-law permitting subscribers to nominate deserving recipients of their personal charity for free care in return for the subscriber's cash donation to the hospital. For example, local employers were offered the right to nominate their employees for free maintenance up to the value of a $25 corporate donation to the hospital. Church groups and fraternal societies could nominate needy members for up to three months of free care in return for a subscription of $25. In 1897 the privilege was extended to members of the hospital trust themselves, who, by purchasing a $5 rather than a $2 annual membership, could claim a

## 42 'A Necessity Among Us'

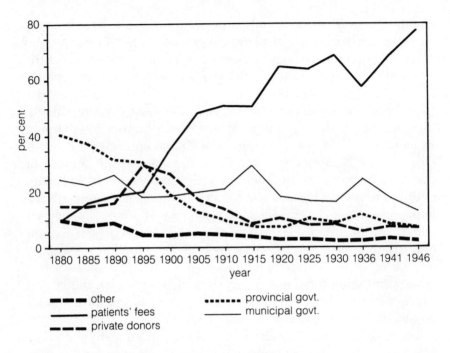

Figure 2. Contributions to total annual income by source, Ontario public general hospitals, 1880–1946

month's free care.[16] Equally effective were the collection boxes installed on the Canadian Pacific's five steamers and voluntarily monitored by the ships' officers.[17] Together with the incidental cash donations of individual citizens and the proceeds of entertainments sponsored by church and cultural groups, these enterprises yielded, in a good year, more than 40 per cent of the hospital's income.

Nor was cash the only resource the community had to offer its hospital. The board actively solicited and received gifts in kind to augment, in particular, the hospital's housekeeping budget. One month's private donations (regularly itemized in the *Times* to thank and encourage donors) included 10 pounds of honey, 4 quarts of grape jelly, 4 quarts of strawberries, 2 quarts of peach preserves, 1 quart of cherries, 1 copy of *The Adventures of Henry M. Stanley*, and a map of the Dominion of Canada.[18] Local merchants were another source of essential supplies – cutlery, dry goods, tableware, and kitchenware – donated partly as a civic responsibility, partly in the expectation of acquiring the hospital's custom.[19] All of this activity was superintended until 1903 by the House Committee, which largely comprised the leadership of the moribund Ladies' Hospital Aid who had been seconded to serve as non-voting members of the committee. In 1903 the board formally invited the women of Owen Sound to create a new Ladies' Auxiliary specifically to assist a reconstituted house committee by raising funds for, offering advice on, and undertaking projects related to the domestic upkeep and improvement of the hospital.[20] Thereafter, much of the G&M's ad hoc solicitation of goods and services was incorporated into the formal activities of the auxiliary, such as Hospital Day, which was initiated in 1904 to focus the donation of in-kind gifts on a single public event.

However, voluntary donations were at best a tenuous source of support. Popular enthusiasm for the hospital cause waxed and waned with the vagaries of the local economy. In at least one respect the hospital paid a significant price for its relentless insistence that it was a charitable enterprise dependent on charity for the perpetuation of its good work: pay patients persistently refused to pay. By 1904 the problem had become so acute that the board secretary's stipend was doubled to enable him to become its bill collector as well.[21] The secretary, Colonel J.P. Telford, was no shrinking violet when it came to protecting the interests of the hospital. When a man whose dog had killed and eaten two of the hospital's chickens balked at paying for their replacements, Telford threatened to recover the loss by having the chickens surgically removed from the dog's stomach.[22] But even Col. Telford's persistence went unrewarded in the face of public indifference to repeated dunning; indifference turned to outright hostility when the board reluctantly placed these bad debts in the hands of a professional credit agency.[23]

From the board's point of view, the most reliable sources of an adequate income ought to have been the municipalities whose citizens, especially their indigent citizens, were the hospital's usual and largest clientele. The board's constant objective was to secure from each of these political constituencies not only annual subscription fees to guarantee the admission of indigent patients to the hospital on the town mayor's, county warden's, or a township reeve's recommendation, but as well annual grants-in-aid of the G&M's general operations.[24] Waiting upon town, county, and township councils was to become one of the most important responsibilities of successive generations of board presidents, who were successful, by and large, in maintaining good working relationships with the local politicians. But the hospital was only one among the long lists of annual supplicants for support from the municipalities' limited tax bases, and although a fairly predictable pattern of municipal support gradually evolved, it was inevitably subject to sudden reversals. The participating township councils limited their contributions to the minimum subscription fees consistent with their residents' historical usage of the hospital. Over a 30-year period these fees never exceeded collectively more than $225 in annual revenue for the hospital. But the senior county administration also negotiated annual grants to the hospital, primarily for the maintenance of indigent county patients. These grants ranged from $200 to $500 until 1908, when the county council agreed, after making no contribution for two years, to raise its annual grant to $1000, partly reflecting the hospital's increased costs and partly to purchase the right to send more free patients to the G&M. Owen Sound's town council, whose constituents made the greatest use of the hospital, usually provided annual grants no larger than those made by Grey County, although they were given more consistently. Most important, both councils tended to respond with greater generosity when other sources of income, particularly private donations, flagged in relation to the hospital's routinely occurring need to increase its operating revenues;[25] both the town and county councils were important sources of capital grants when the expansion of the hospital's physical facilities became a pressing necessity after 1905.

As its annual balance sheets indicate, between 1893 and 1918 the hospital trust always operated within the restrictive limits of budgets in which expenditure was simply a function of income. There was no room for advanced fiscal planning in an enterprise preoccupied with its monthly cash flow and in which the operations of the hospital were subject to sudden and unplanned changes as the result of unanticipated shortfalls in monthly income. In the beginning the hospital's average operating costs per patient-day were nearly one dollar (see Table 1). Experience and greater institutional efficiency soon reduced these expenditures to less than 70 cents for the remainder of the decade, but the return of general prosperity at the beginning of the new century and the rapidly growing demand for the hospital's services conspired nearly to double total annual operating costs between 1902 and 1908. In the next four years they rose by another 50 per cent. In one way or another income not only had to keep pace with these operating expenses, but had to provide essential surpluses for capital projects, equipment upgrading, and debt servicing. Throughout the period the provincial government's subsidy was fixed at 30 cents per patient day for indigent patients, in effect falling in value from 50 per cent of the cost of maintaining an indigent in 1900 to less than 25 per cent in 1910. The hospital's other sources of revenue had to provide the difference in addition to meeting the operating expenses associated with its routine activities; hence the constant lobbying for increased municipal grants, and, as time passed, the board's preoccupation with the fees charged to paying patients, the relative proportion of beds occupied by paying patients, and the quality of the hospital's services and environment in relation to the preferences of a clientele now willing and able to pay for something more than basic care. Catering to these new interests produced additional revenue but led in turn to increased costs, and the problem came full circle. Not surprisingly, over the years the board of trustees became especially adept at crisis management.

The hospital's major expenses were wages, food, housekeeping supplies, drugs (primarily alcohol) and medical supplies, fuel, and building maintenance. Wherever possible, successive boards introduced economies to control these expenses in the long term, and when these strategies failed implemented drastic measures to head off disaster in the short term. A policy initiated with the inception of the hospital was the decision to raise at least some of its food supply on its four acres of land, which eventually supported a vegetable garden, an orchard, a flock of chickens, and the hospital cow. These arrangements, however, merely augmented the food the hospital was compelled to buy from local merchants at prices that began to rise dramatically after 1900, as did the cost of the coal and wood the hospital burned for fuel. By 1904 the board was inviting tenders for the contracts for the hospital's annual meat, grocery, dairy produce, wood and coal supplies (and invariably accepting the lowest bids) and buying its cleaning and laundry supplies in bulk from Toronto wholesalers.[26]

The board's wage bill proved less tractable. Hospitals are essentially labour-intensive enterprises, and as the G&M's business increased it became necessary to hire more staff, especially graduate nurses, who tended to be greatly overworked during the hospital's periods of peak activity and underemployed at other times. Twice between 1895 and 1904 the lady superintendent was specifically ordered to send her nurses out to private homes in order to raise additional income for the hospital during periods of financial crisis.[27] But this was probably a common practice, given the town's historical shortage of private nurses and the hospital's invariably fragile monthly balances. The seasonality of demand for nursing services at the G&M was always compounded by the preference among graduate nurses for private duty or for employment in a large institution where salaries were higher and career opportunities, either as nursing instructors or supervisors, were greater. Even lady superintendents (of whom there were six in the G&M between 1893 and 1912) were part of a highly mobile workforce moving around the province's, and Canada's, rapidly expanding system of general hospitals in search of professional advancement. They customarily stayed at the G&M for about five years. For all of these reasons the G&M's board of trustees concluded, in 1900, that a training school for nurses would be a useful adjunct to the hospital. The labour of student nurses would reduce the hospital's wage bill, create a dependable labour supply for both hospital and home nursing, provide an inducement for some graduate nurses (including lady superintendents) to remain at the G&M, generate income for the hospital, and 'enhance the standing and prestige' of the G&M among its sister institutions in southern Ontario.[28]

Since there were no provincial regulations governing the creation of such schools, their curricula, or the standards of competence required for the certification of their graduates, the board was free to advertise for probationers immediately. Six young women who met the requirements for admission – at least 20 years old and 'quick and bright and possessed of a good high school education'[29] – subsequently comprised the first class, which began its two-year (increased to three years beginning with the class of 1905) training program in May 1901. They followed a curriculum devised by the medical staff, who also served as the instructors in obstetrics, gynecology, pediatrics, surgery, anatomy and physiology, medicine, and hygiene. The matron was responsible for the courses in general nursing.[30] The first graduation exercises in November 1903 celebrated training 'that brings out all of the kindest traits of womankind.'[31] There were other, more practical reasons for thanksgiving. The students performed all of the duties of graduate nurses, albeit under supervision, effectively doubling the hospital's labour force at less than half the cost of hiring a comparable number of graduate nurses.

In implementing the program for these purposes, the G&M was not alone. In both Canada and the United States, nursing schools increasingly solved the problem of guaranteeing the availability of an inexpensive but more or less adequately trained workforce with the characteristics that hospitals required and patients admired – efficiency, obedience, a working knowledge of the principles of antisepsis, a general understanding of the scientific basis of medical treatment,[32] and, above all, selfless dedication to the welfare of patients combined with an iron constitution, the better to withstand six-and-a-half days per week of 12-hour shifts followed by classes.[33] Not yet a self-defining or self-regulating profession, nursing, except in very large teaching hospitals, still reflected the paternalistic interests of lay trustees, the absolute authority of lady superintendents in the workplace, and the expectations of patients for whom nurses were often, at best, highly qualified domestic servants. Still, as the journalist Sara Jeanette Duncan observed of the Toronto General's graduating class of 1886, 'the social condition of nurses [was] vastly different from what it used to be' just a few years before when 'the profession had little dignity and few rewards' compared to the importance now attached to the services of 'a well brought up class of Canadian women' trained as professional nurses.³⁴

The board's escalating labour, food, and fuel costs, in addition to its mortgages and its debt collection problems, left little enough surplus income from any source to improve the G&M's physical facilities or upgrade its medical technology. As late as 1900 the hospital's operating-room was still lit by coal oil lanterns, much to the dismay of the inspector who recommended the installation, if not of electric lights, at least of safer gas lighting. The conversion to gas was finally made in 1901, but until 1911, when electrical service was installed in conjunction with the construction of the new wing, lighting levels were still inadequate for any sort of surgery past mid-afternoon, thereby restricting the hospital's effectiveness as an emergency treatment facility.³⁵ More pressing necessities were an ice house and a new laundry, both essential prerequisites for the health of convalescing patients. Both were constructed by the board only after agonizing debates over the wisdom of increasing the trust's debt load.³⁶ The only other major improvement, the construction of two verandas as solaria for patients, was a project initiated by the Ladies' Auxiliary and paid for by their fund-raising enterprises, which increasingly relieved the board of expenses associated with the hospital's housekeeping and minor maintenance needs. But by 1909 even the goodwill of the auxiliary had become exhausted by conditions that the medical staff, the lady superintendent, the nurses, and the public found intolerable. In June the ladies made their case bluntly. The hospital was 'not up to the required standard' and unless the board agreed to rectify the 'deplorable' situation immediately, the volunteers would waste no more energy on the G&M. A month later the board agreed to a plan to expand and modernize the hospital.³⁷

What was wrong with the General and Marine hospital in 1909 constituted a catalogue of deficiencies that had accumulated over a period of about five years, roughly since the hospital entered its second decade of operations. Many of these deficiencies were the result of physical deterioration and operating inefficiencies simply attributable to the trust's tenuous financial history, compounded by the cautious fiscal policies pursued by the board on which the hospital's major creditor, the Grey and Bruce Savings and Loan Company, was overrepresented. Some of the problems were attributable to the need to rely on in-kind charitable contributions instead of being able to purchase more durable goods and equipment. But many of the G&M's perceived shortcomings were liabilities only in relation to a growing wish list of desirable innovations, representing the rapidly developing concept of the modern medical centre, compiled by a variety of participants in the process.

The hospital's medical staff, for example, had begun to lobby for the expansion and upgrading of the hospital in 1904, arguing that increasing the hospital's capacity to accommodate more surgical cases and more complex surgery was consistent with its necessary transition from a custodial facility to a modern centre for the treatment of disease. By 1909 the doctors' discontentment was also focused on the quality of convalescent care, the professional standards of the nursing staff, the competence of the lady superintendent, and the priorities of the board. The board, they claimed, valued economy ahead of efficient medical care and encouraged the lady superintendent to provide the cheapest food, drugs, and supplies instead of the more expensive but more effective dietary provisions, pharmaceuticals, and medical supplies recommended by physicians. The matron stood accused of being 'unable to carry out ... up-to-date scientific surgical techniques or to teach her nurses the same,' especially the principles of antiseptic surgery, with the result that her nurse trainees were deemed by the physicians to be unfit for employment at the G&M or anywhere else. Finally, the lack of any staff member trained in the science of dietetics meant that convalescing patients could not receive the dietary therapy now considered essential by their physicians.[38]

These criticisms reflected, in a general sense, the Canadian medical fraternity's growing vested interest in the hospital as their preferred workplace where they not only dispensed medical charity on behalf of the community but, in return, earned the right to treat their private patients in an environment compatible with their scientific imperative and conducive to the needs and demands of a paying clientele. As the *Canadian Lancet* repeatedly insisted, hospitals 'should take special pains to safeguard the interests of the medical profession,' should be centres of 'scientific good work and of professional good feeling,' and should 'do nothing that would deprive a practitioner of a fee.'[39] Bad science, bad food, and sloppy nursing care left the G&M culpable on all three fronts from the physicians' perspective. The lady superintendent, Jessie Duncan, promptly resigned, undoubtedly mystified by the litany of incompetence directed at her after five years of promoting many of the same objectives desired by the physicians. A diet kitchen, an adequate staff of graduate nurses and trained orderlies, less crowded public wards, and adequate housing for nurses compelled to live in conditions worse than they encountered during long shifts, 'among all classes of people, in the hospital and in private homes' were high on her list of improvements necessary to modernize the hospital.[40] In these matters she had the unequivocal support of the Ladies' Auxiliary, who, in addition to their lengthy inventory of the G&M's general deficiencies, had already made a nurses' home, an isolated obstetrical ward and nursery, and optional private accommodations for maternity cases their particular hobby-horses after 1904.

To these specific innovations must be added one more: vastly expanded accommodations for private and semi-private patients. By 1904 this expanding clientele of paying patients tended to insist on the preferential accommodation and care represented by the G&M's private rooms and semi-private wards. As demand began to exceed the supply of facilities for these patients, the board of trustees was quick to recognize the income-generating potential of full-pay patients in terms of both preferred care and surcharges for certain hospital services. The operating-room charges implemented in 1907 were simply a foretaste of the board's decision a year later to double its charges for private rooms and to increase rates for semi-private accommodation by 80 per cent.[41] But what the board had to offer in return was a hospital its friends, employees, advisers, and patrons considered to be an outmoded and inadequate setting for the practice of modern medicine and the care of paying patients.

The initial impetus to develop a plan for expanding and modernizing the General and Marine Hospital was the medical staff's petition, submitted in December 1904, urging the board of trustees to raise $15,000 immediately for the necessary improvements. The following April, the board, after lengthy discussions, agreed to act on the recommendation; but another 18 months passed before a general plan of a new wing, with its price-tag of $30,000, was presented to board members.[42] No record survives of the discussions which evidently convinced the board to delay further action on the plan, but a number of circumstances may have contributed to the members' reluctance to move ahead. The most obvious problem was the G&M's continuing financial crisis resulting primarily from its perennial cash flow difficulties exacerbated by mounting expenditures for the maintenance of its outdated, deteriorating physical plant and for additional housekeeping and supervisory staff in consequence of its heavier patient loads. As monthly deficits piled up, the board became preoccupied with these problems, even to the point of implementing wage freezes and investigating the rate of gas consumption in the nurses' residence in order to save money.[43] Under these conditions, planning for a major expansion was at best an exercise in wishful thinking. It also seems, however, that the board of trustees took a calculated risk in agreeing to allow one of its own members to undertake a private fund-raising campaign in support of a major program of expansion. In April 1907, W.H. Smith offered to raise $50,000 for the trust independently. His assurances were sufficiently convincing that a year passed before the board began to inquire about the success of Smith's campaign and the whereabouts of the subscriptions he claimed to have collected. They amounted in the end to $377.60, and a year of valuable planning time was lost.[44] Whatever the cause, in the spring of 1909 these repeated delays finally galvanized the Ladies' Auxiliary into doing their 'duty,' in spite, they said, of the board's long history of 'completely ignor[ing]' their advice. This time the board listened.[45]

Preliminary architectural drawings were ready within a month, and when the board reconvened in the autumn, the members of the trust approved its recommendation that the Ladies' Auxiliary and the medical staff should be granted representation (by nomination) on the board in order to facilitate planning for the new hospital.[46] The winter months were spent finalizing the plans, which were formally approved in June 1910. They involved construction of a new wing to include a nurses' residence; modern operating suites; a dispensary; surgical, medical, and obstetrical wards; apartments for the lady superintendent; and a doctor's room. As well, the interior of the original building was to be remodelled, and in both wings the most advanced construction methods and up-to-date appliances and equipment were to be installed, following the recommendations of Dr Middlebro, who undertook an extensive tour of American hospitals to document the state of the art of hospital construction. The total cost was set at $30,000, of which basic new construction represented about $15,000.[47] A month later contracts were signed with the builders, and the corner-stone was laid on the 24th of August. Henceforward, the G&M was to be known as the Owen Sound and Grey County General and Marine Hospital to acknowledge its regional mandate and, just as important, its regional base of essential financial and political support.[48]

Considering its longstanding anxieties about the hospital's precarious financial situation and the miserable failure of Smith's one-man fund-raising campaign, the board had every reason to be concerned about the added financial burden represented by the new wing and the public's response to a plea for subscriptions to underwrite the costs of construction. Consequently, before giving final approval for the project the board had written to John D. Rockefeller, arguably the richest man in America and its best-known philanthropist, seeking a contribution of $10,000. The board's reasoning seems to have been that with two-thirds of the construction costs of the new wing in hand from a single gift and with a prior guarantee of up to $7000 in mortgage financing from the Trader's Bank for the remaining third, at least the basic costs of construction could be met without depending on the unpredictable outcome of a public appeal.[49] When this solicitation brought no response, the board made two decisions. First, no building was to commence until the trust had $20,000 cash on hand to pay for the construction of the new wing. Second, the now inevitable fund-raising campaign would target corporate donors – local, provincial, and national – as the primary source of the required funding and the principal objects of interest to a special committee of canvassers created by the board.[50]

It proved to be a useful strategy. The corporate, small business, and professional solicitation yielded pledges of at least $7800, not far short of the sum requested from Rockefeller, which was soon surpassed when the president of the board, J.M. Kilbourn, and his first vice-president, D.M. Butchart – the Portland cement magnate – made personal gifts of $1000 and $1500 respectively. Four municipal capital grants, $5000 from the Town of Owen Sound, $1000 from Grey County, $500 from Sydenham Township, and $250 from Derby, raised the total amount pledged by business, government, and major private philanthropists to a sum roughly equal to the costs of the new construction.[51] The example set by the major private and public donors seems to have had the desired effect. In the first week of the campaign, launched in mid-June 1910, the committee wrote pledges for about $18,000. By mid-September the total had risen to nearly $20,000, and by the end of the campaign $23,000 in subscriptions had been collected, leaving $7000 of the projected costs of expansion to be financed by mortgage.[52] Among the private citizens who pledged subscriptions, about one-third were residents of the townships surrounding Owen Sound, and a surprisingly large number of individual donations were from the town of Wiarton, the centre of the Bruce Peninsula's lumber industry. In the end, however, it is not the $5000 contributed to the project by ordinary citizens that seems particularly remarkable, but rather the apparent cooperation between the private and public sectors of the local economy in providing roughly 52 per cent of the total financing in the form of 75 per cent of the funds raised through subscriptions. This suggests that business and government no longer considered the hospital to be merely an object of casual charity, but a community resource worth the investment of significant sums of public and private capital. As the president of the board explained to the G&M's graduating nurses shortly after the official opening of the new wing on 25 June 1911: 'This is ... the age of progress. Owen Sound is a progressive town, and there is no better evidence of ... progress ... than the improvement of the facilities for the alleviation of ... suffering.'[53]

The expanded and improved General and Marine Hospital's stock-in-trade, according to the editor of the weekly *Times*, would now be 'efficient work' in 'up-to-date medical science.'[54] This was not merely local boosterism. Even amid the disruptions of the construction project (which was not entirely finished until the early spring of 1912) the 'medical and surgical care of patients [was] equal to that of any other hospital' in Ontario, according to the provincial inspector, who found the G&M to be 'well and carefully managed' and supported by a greater degree of public confidence than at any time in the past.[55] For its part, the board of trustees took considerable satisfaction in having moved the hospital from a state of 'decrepid [sic] age' to one of 'youthful vigour' by constructing 'one of the most modern, complete and well appointed institutions for the care and healing of the sick to be found anywhere.'[56] These improvements had been purchased, nevertheless, at considerable cost in relation to the actual funds available for construction and to the opportunities for recapturing unfunded construction debts and for increasing revenues to meet the higher operating costs associated with expansion. Nursing services, for example, had to be expanded to provide higher staff/patient ratios in the new private, semi-private, and obstetrics wards. An assistant superintendent was required to supervise the operating-rooms; and a housekeeper, with a degree in home economics, was at last employed to supervise the kitchen and domestic staff. With reason, the board continued to worry that the costs of this progress would prove in the end to be too great a burden in relation to the trust's ability to sustain a commitment to a significantly higher order of medical services. Having eliminated the G&M's outstanding mortgaged debt just prior to the construction of the new wing, the board emerged from that exercise faced not only with a new mortgage of nearly $7000, but with a comparable bank loan to meet its increased operating costs and, as revenues dwindled during the pre-war recession, with the loss of the overdraft privileges that had carried the hospital through its recurrent monthly cash flow problems.[57]

Again the nurses were sent out for private duty to raise needed revenues, operating economies were introduced, the ward rates for indigent patients were increased by 40 per cent and the lady superintendent was instructed to collect a week's maintenance in advance from paying patients at the beginning of each week of their stay, and to remove private and semi-private ward patients to the public wards if they failed to pay in advance.[58] There were, however, real limitations on the board's ability to increase operating revenues, to restrain spending, to improve cash flows, and, withal, to satisfy the public's developing expectation that the hospital should be the source of the best medical care available at a price acceptable to its now largely paying clientele. No longer a charity, not yet a business, the hospital was nevertheless a service already deemed essential to all classes of the population. It seemed to the board to fit more neatly the definition of those other services – public transportation, electrification, sanitation, waterworks, telephone systems – which, under the leadership of a vigorous North American urban reform movement, increasingly were being redefined as public rather than private utilities to be owned, funded, and operated by the community in the interests of all of its citizens.[59] Amidst the fiscal aftermath of its effort to make the General and Marine Hospital a monument to the promises of the new science of medicine, the board prayed that 'the burden of maintaining this absolutely necessary branch of Public Utility' would soon be relieved 'by a general taxation to be collected as [are] monies for other municipal requirements as the most equitable and easy method' of providing hospital services to all members of the community.[60]

This perception of the hospital as an institution at a critical juncture, on the eve of the First World War, in its necessary evolution from a public charity to a municipal public utility was widespread, at least among hospital trustees and administrators. In just 20 years their priorities had moved relentlessly from the medical recovery of indigent and homeless patients to the fiscal recovery of apparently uncontrollable operating costs by providing at substantial prices the services the hospital once offered free of charge. Vastly increased public support, especially from municipal tax bases, was becoming one of their favourite themes, particularly as the provincial government edged closer, in 1912, to a sweeping revision of its hospital legislation. But the expectation that government – local, provincial, or federal – would find in public hospitals an irresistible object of increased public support was, in 1912, contrary to both the nature of government and the established facts of hospital economics everywhere in North America. The modern hospital, in its first manifestation, was manifestly an enterprise whose immediate success would depend on the public's willingness and ability to pay the full costs of a now highly desirable commodity.

By 1914 the first stage of the Owen Sound and Grey County General and Marine Hospital's transition from a medical charity to a modern health care centre was complete. The essential hallmarks of that transition were: the growing primacy of surgery and, to a lesser extent, obstetrics within the hospital; the expansion of the hospital's clientele to include all classes of the population and, in more equitable proportions, both sexes; the shift in the hospital's admission priorities and in the use of its resources from charity cases to paying patients; the developing institutional emphasis on cost effectiveness and cost recovery in the face of rapidly escalating health care delivery costs; and, finally, public recognition of the hospital as a socially and medically indispensable institution. In these respects, the G&M's historical development was not different from the experience of other public general hospitals founded in the late nineteenth century as secular charities and subjected to the complex processes of social change and scientific innovation that characterized the quarter-century prior to the First World War. What seems remarkable is that these processes appear to have produced, at different times and in quite disparate locales throughout North America, fundamentally the same types of institutions pursuing similar strategies to solve common problems and to achieve common objectives. By 1912 the G&M was part of an emerging health care 'system.'

# 3

## 'Once a Patient, Always a Booster': Standardization and Stability, 1914–29

The newly transformed Owen Sound and Grey County General and Marine Hospital and the new Toronto General Hospital both opened their doors in 1912. There, at first glance, the similarity ends. The Toronto General's medical, surgical, obstetrical, pathology, immunology, emergency, outpatient, x-ray, and housekeeping departments floated on indestructible battleship linoleum tastefully matched with their scrubbable pastel walls and vitreous china fixtures. Hospital equipment moved around the General's 10 acres of covered space on newly designed silent rubber wheels. One hundred and fifty private patients lived en suite in rooms designed to overcome the 'deadly sameness' of institutional architecture. Any patient could summon a nurse instantly with a bedside 'silent call' button, just as departments and nursing stations were linked by a silent telephone system. Sterilized chilled water coursed through special lines to drinking fountains on each floor. Twelve operating suites were available to accommodate the hospital's teaching function. Nurses and nursing students occupied single rooms, ate in a modern dining hall set aside for them and medical students, and took classes in specially equipped lecture halls and demonstration laboratories. The General's self-contained power plant generated 1850 horsepower to drive the hospital's equipment. A massive incinerator disposed of all of the hospital's garbage. The hospital included none of 'the fads which are so striking a feature in some institutions': it merely 'possess[ed] everything that is regarded as necessary.'[1]

By these standards, the refurbished G&M left much to be desired as a temple of scientific medicine and modern hospital service. Its three small balconies were pale reflections of the General's roof-top solaria. Its three services – medical, surgical, and obstetric – enjoyed only the distinction of nominal separation. The G&M had no laboratory, x-ray, or hydrotherapy facilities. Its obstetrics ward lacked privacy. Its steam laundry, morgue, and ice-house were as antiquated as the General's combined powerhouse/refrigeration unit/electrically powered laundry were ultra-modern. Apart from its lighting, the only electrical conveniences in the G&M were its elevator and (non-silent) call bell system, both installed to ease the burden of its largely student nursing staff who lived in cramped quarters, did their lessons after their 12 hour shifts, and learned their craft not in demonstration rooms, but at the patient's bedside. Still, the G&M boasted two up-to-date operating-rooms and the best surgical equipment available. Every floor was served by a special diet kitchen, a dispensary, and modern bathroom and lavatory facilities (the conversion to indoor conveniences did not get into full sway in Owen Sound itself until 1914).[2] The newest private accommodations included fireplaces, bathrooms, and furnishings which contemporary observers described as extravagant; even the public wards were regarded as concessions to the physical and mental comfort of patients within the context of an institution which was heralded as 'the latest and most advanced' expression of modern hospital construction.[3]

In fact, the General and the G&M represented only differences in degree, not in kind. Each in its respective pursuit of modernity had acquired in the eyes of both external observers and of those who worked on behalf of or who were residents in the hospital a new social and medical legitimacy largely divorced from the hospital's historical identity as a charity. The relative significance of the various factors which contributed to that new legitimacy is still open to debate. Certainly the range and the efficacy of hospital-centred medical therapeutics left much to be desired whether the patient was treated by the Toronto General's expert consultants or the

G&M's less qualified medical staff. Surgery, however effective as a radical treatment for certain discrete diseases, was nevertheless limited to a rather narrow spectrum of life-threatening or acute illnesses and injuries. Recent advances in immunology and serology had produced new weapons for the war on some bacterial organisms, diphtheria for example, while the emerging science of pharmaceutical chemistry had begun to develop synthetic drugs to control pain and fever more effectively.[4] But most degenerative diseases were no more amenable to treatment by modern medical science than they had been in the hands of the bleeding, purging, and blistering physicians of the nineteenth century, and the era of wonder drugs with which to treat disease-bearing micro-organisms had not yet arrived. Even as late as the 1930s the G&M's inventory of drugs consisted of about equal parts of synthetic pain-killers and traditional remedies – cascara, licorice, sodium bromide, quinine, asafetida, eucalyptus compound, cocaine, calomel – and not much else.[5] In an era in which the leading causes of premature death – tuberculosis, the annual ravages of water-borne diseases, and cholera infantum – were largely environmentally induced, hospital-based medicine was almost irrelevant compared to the challenges still facing the public health system.[6] The momentous decline in Ontario's death rate between 1900 and 1940, with the exception of maternal mortality and deaths from appendicitis and peritonitis, was principally the result of public health rather than medical activity.[7]

Apparently, the transformation of the public general hospital from a charitable institution to the seat of 'scientific' medicine for the entire community, whether in Owen Sound or elsewhere, was the product of limited, yet powerful forces. The first of these was the medical profession itself. Owen Sound doctors were no longer content with their image as 'country' doctors clinically confined by the limitations of their surgeries or their patients' homes. The ability to manage, or at least supervise, the course of acute illnesses with the assistance of trained, competent personnel in a setting conducive to convalescence and recovery (hence the dispute with Miss Duncan over drugs, diet therapy, and antisepsis) was as much a part of the therapeutic 'revolution' that now distinguished scientific medicine from its 'irregular' competition – quacks – as the new accuracy of the surgeon's scalpel. Just as important, the middle class, both as paying consumers of health care and as the town's perpetual civic boosters, supported and promoted these developments as essential to the whole community's well-being. One commentator retrospectively placed the effort to fund and build the new hospital in the same category, in terms of social commitment and financial generosity, as the patriotic voluntarism that swept over Owen Sound between 1914 and 1916.[8] This suggests, in the absence of other evidence, that a transformation had also taken place in social perceptions of disease, the promise of scientifically approved therapeutics, and, in particular, the benefits of institutionally based health care. It was a case, as with so much of the history of modern health care, of rising public expectations stimulated by the often more apparent than real pace of medical progress.

A third force in this transition was the growing influence of a new breed of professional hospital administrators and planners. For example, *The Hospital World*, the first major journal for hospital administrators, was launched in 1912 with a catalogue of the questions that 'hospital workers the world over' needed to resolve. Who should pay for hospitals? Where should hospitals be located? How should hospital services be internally structured? Should rich and poor be treated under the same roof? Should patients disrobe in the admitting department or the ward? What was the most appropriate flooring for hospitals? Did doctors, laymen, or nurses make the best superintendents? What was the optimum size for an operating-room? Should hospital practice be restricted to specialists or open to all physicians? Was the patient a 'person' or a 'case,' and what was the effect of creeping 'institutionalism' on the patient's 'real self'? The editors of the journal suggested that it would take generations to sort out the most appropriate answers to 'these and scores of other subjects' relevant to the advent of the modern hospital.[9]

Among these questions, the most urgent was who should pay for the proliferation of hospitals required to meet public demand for hospital-centred treatment employing the latest advances in medical science and technology. The president of the Canadian Hospital Association (founded in 1906 to provide a forum for administrators and trustees) accurately predicted the outcome of the hospital revolution, one of the 'great reforms of modern times':

> Antiseptic and aseptic surgery [have] ushered in a new era ... Step by step patients have been gaining confidence in hospitals ... Thousands of hospitals have been erected ... during the last few years ... The end is not yet [in sight]. The end of this century will mark an enormous increase in the number of institutions for the care of the sick ... In order to maintain this ever increasing number of institutions, larger and still larger sums of money will be needed. This will necessitate the educating of the people ... into more liberal support of hospitals ... If hospitals are to advance and keep up their present standard of efficiency there must be more money forthcoming ... [T]here must be a mighty awakening of public conscience in order that ... [we may] come into our rightful inheritance.[10]

He concluded that the hospital revolution could succeed only through the active participation of provincial and municipal governments and private citizens as the principal benefactors of hospitals, which would earn increased public trust as much through managerial efficiency as therapeutic efficacy. Organization, systematization, vigilance, and cost effectiveness were the handmaidens of productivity, the ultimate measure of value for money invested.

The assumption that private philanthropy would continue to be an important source of funding for public hospitals was already open to question. However significant in absolute terms, private donations and subscriptions represented a rapidly declining proportion of total hospital income and tended to be both solicited and designated for capital projects. Increasingly, patients' fees and government grants accounted for the bulk of hospital operating revenues in Ontario (see Figure 1), and it was ultimately on the generosity of the public purse that the hospital reformers pinned their hopes for the coming revolution in patient care. Hence their initial enthusiasm for the Ontario government's Act Relating to Hospitals and Charitable Institutions (RSO 1897, c. 320, s. 1) which was proclaimed on 16 April 1912.

The Hospital and Charitable Institutions Act updated and revised earlier legislation that had made provision for the incorporation, inspection, and funding (through per diem grants for eligible patients) of public hospitals in the province. In particular, the revised legislation introduced one reform much sought after by hospitals. It rendered municipalities legally liable for the costs of maintaining their indigent citizens in hospital, fixed the extent of their liability at $7.00 per patient per week, and placed the onus on municipalities to prove that indigents admitted for treatment were not their responsibility (cl. 23). In effect the legislation promised to bring to an end the public hospitals' annual pilgrimages to city, town, and county councils to negotiate voluntary grants for the maintenance of municipal indigents, and to provide hospitals with a calculable income related in some way to their costs for maintaining non-paying patients, always a significant proportion of their clientele.

The editors of *The Hospital World* heralded this legislation as a 'splendid bill' embodying the 'most advanced legislation ever introduced in Canada,' not least of all because it also gave public hospitals the power of expropriation and initiated a provincial registry of nurses who were graduates of training schools established in government-assisted public hospitals.[11] But the identification of 'registered' nurses, a licence to expand, and guaranteed income from the treatment of indigent patients could have been interpreted just as easily as carrots on the long stick of government regulation. The act also required hospitals to admit any patient who presented himself for treatment, including tubercular patients (only patients with placardable communicable diseases were excluded). Similarly, the act denied provincial subventions for paying patients to all hospitals in receipt of provincial grants-in-aid for more than 10 years. Since the act defined a *paying patient* as any person who paid, or had paid on his behalf from non-government sources, more for his treatment than the indigent rate of $7.00 per week (cl. 6), the legislation had the effect of depressing public ward rates in established hospitals if those institutions wished to continue to preserve the eligibility of their part-pay patients (usually the working poor) or, for that matter, any paying public ward patient for provincial subsidies. Those subsidies, together with the new municipal rate, represented about 85 per cent of the average costs of maintaining one patient for one day in a typical public general hospital in Ontario in 1912. The unfunded costs had to be raised from other sources, presumably through higher fees charged to private ward patients, but the legislation restricted the hospitals' freedom in this respect as well. No provincial grant could be claimed by any hospital whose total annual operating income (not including the provincial grant) exceeded its annual operating costs (cl. 4). On balance, the new Hospitals and Charitable Institutions Act was a significant improvement over its predecessors; but in the developing field of hospital care, events were moving at a faster pace than legislation could anticipate.

This was the context within which the newly expanded and refurbished General and Marine Hospital sought to fulfil its mandate as a community health care centre between the Great War and the Great Depression. As remote as it was from the battlefields of Europe, Owen Sound, like other communities on the home front, was affected by the conflict in a variety of ways that were reflected in the operations of the hospital. The war effort increasingly diverted money, labour, and goods from the community as the Canadian government geared the nation to wage total war on Germany. Still saddled with a significant debt from its program of expansion, the board of trustees found itself, after 1914, in double fiscal jeopardy – unable to compete with war-related charities for donations and faced with rapidly inflating costs for goods and services. The board calculated that between 1913 and 1917 the hospital's operating costs increased 52 per cent. In fact, between the beginning and the end of the war, as Table 5 reveals, the hospital's operating costs doubled while the annual number of patient days increased by only about 60 per cent, with no commensurate increases in municipal or provincial grants. In 1915 the president of the board, F.W. Harrison (whose family was one of the G&M's greatest benefactors), frankly admitted that '[u]nder the present conditions, it [was] useless to refer to the ... urgent needs of the Hospital' in the hope of tapping public generosity.[13] The board had no choice but to tighten its belt wherever economies could be made, and to authorize only those new expenditures essential to the hospital's ability to function. Consequently, in 1915 (and again in 1917) the board implemented a hiring freeze which extended even to the admission of additional

TABLE 5
Summary statistics, G&M Hospital, 1915–29

|  | Year ending 30 September | | | | | | | |
| --- | --- | --- | --- | --- | --- | --- | --- | --- |
|  | 1915 | 1917 | 1919 | 1921 | 1923 | 1925 | 1927 | 1929 |
| No. of patients treated* | 474 | 467 | 737 | 824 | 835 | 814 | 976 | 1,226 |
| Total patient days | 6,998 | 7,065 | 11,141 | 12,671 | 11,133 | 11,244 | 12,696 | 16,490 |
| Average stay | 14.8 | 15.1 | 15.1 | 15.4 | 13.30 | 13.8 | 13.0 | 13.5 |
| Total operating income ($) | 13,957.07 | 16,672.39 | 28,174.07 | 36,142.17 | 35,018.85 | 31,727.58 | 38,517.47 | 50,352.70 |
| Municipal grants ($) | 3,035.00 | 3,306.00 | 4,100.00 | 3,050.00 | 4,500.00 | 2,066.50 | 3,078.68 | 500.00 |
| % of income | 21.7 | 19.8 | 14.6 | 8.4 | 12.9 | 6.5 | 8.0 | 1.0 |
| Provincial grants ($) | 652.60 | 486.43 | 975.11 | 2,094.30 | 2,268.80 | 2,063.90 | 2,398.30 | 3,133.50 |
| % of income | 4.7 | 2.9 | 3.5 | 5.8 | 6.5 | 6.6 | 6.2 | 6.2 |
| Subscriptions ($) | 632.76 | 357.95 | 2,434.74 | 3,058.05 | 4,177.99 | 3,868.60 | 5,255.00 | 300.00 |
| % of income | 4.5 | 2.1 | 8.6 | 8.5 | 11.9 | 12.2 | 13.6 | 0.6 |
| Patient fees ($) | 9,636.71 | 12,522.01 | 20,664.22 | 27,851.82 | 24,072.06 | 23,728.58 | 27,855.49 | 46,419.20 |
| % of income | 69.0 | 75.1 | 73.3 | 77.1 | 68.7 | 74.8 | 72.3 | 92.2 |
| Total operating costs ($) | 13,052.12 | 18,061.13 | 26,353.40 | 33,818.96 | 32,506.25 | 31,766.23 | 36,295.59 | 47,421.25 |
| Cost of food ($) | 4,317.57 | 6,353.03 | 9,883.73 | 11,901.35 | 10,248.29 | 10,138.01 | 12,861.41 | 13,056.67 |
| % of costs | 33.1 | 35.2 | 37.5 | 35.2 | 31.5 | 31.9 | 35.4 | 27.5 |
| Supplies and services ($) | 8,734.55 | 11,708.10 | 16,469.67 | 21,917.61 | 22,257.96 | 21,628.22 | 23,434.18 | 34,364.58 |
| % of costs | 66.9 | 64.8 | 62.5 | 64.8 | 68.5 | 68.1 | 64.6 | 72.5 |
| Patient fees as % of operating costs | 73.8 | 69.3 | 78.4 | 82.4 | 74.1 | 74.7 | 76.7 | 97.9 |
| Municipal & provincial grants as % of operating costs | 28.3 | 21.0 | 19.3 | 15.2 | 20.8 | 13.0 | 15.1 | 7.7 |

| | | | | | | | | |
|---|---|---|---|---|---|---|---|---|
| Patient fees & grants as % of total operating costs | 102.1 | 90.3 | 97.7 | 97.6 | 94.9 | 87.7 | 91.8 | 105.5 |
| Income per patient day | 1.99 | 2.36 | 2.53 | 2.85 | 3.15 | 2.82 | 3.03 | 3.05 |
| Cost per patient day | 1.87 | 2.56 | 2.37 | 2.67 | 2.92 | 2.83 | 2.86 | 2.88 |
| Usage (% of capacity) | 44.6 | 45.0 | 71.0 | 80.7 | 70.9 | 71.6 | 72.5 | 94.1 |
| No. of surgical cases | 284 | 336 | 455 | 576 | | 604 | | 623 |

*Excludes newborns
SOURCES: Sessional Papers of Ontario; Annual Reports, G&M Hospital

nursing students. To preserve existing nursing positions the senior nursing staff took a voluntary cut in salary, and the hospital's rates were raised once again (which had the undesired effect of dampening both admissions and the length of patient stays).[14] By 1916 the board was nevertheless faced with the necessity of either improving its maternity/obstetric service by providing greater privacy or losing the hospital's accreditation. This involved moving the maternity ward from the second floor (which it shared with the surgical ward) to the third floor. The move apparently created a new flurry of interest in hospital births among women, who also demanded private or semi-private rooms and special nursing services (see Figure 2). The result was to skew limited resources towards the obstetrics service at a time when the hospital was under increased pressure from other quarters.[15]

In 1916 the 147th and 248th battalions were training in Grey County and the G&M's facilities were used by the Canadian Army Medical Corps, which had to grapple with a major outbreak of typhoid fever in the camp in addition to the casualties – normal as well as extraordinary – generated by a large concentration of men engaged in intensive training manoeuvres.[16] The strain placed on the hospital's resources, especially its surgical capacity, by the presence of 'The Greys' nevertheless paled into insignificance in comparison with the war-induced outbreak of 'Spanish Influenza' that gripped Owen Sound in 1918. In spite of its name, the virus was introduced into the trenches of Europe by Chinese labourers employed by the British army. It spread quickly among the troops at the front and was soon transmitted to army camps in England and was then transported to North America by returning soldiers. The virus and its carriers fanned out across the country along the major transportation arteries until, by October 1918, Canadians everywhere had fallen victims to the world-wide pandemic of a particularly virulent strain of influenza characterized by abnormally high mortality rates, especially among 20–40-year-olds.[17]

Owen Sound's experience with the 'Spanish flu' was a microcosm of the effects of the pandemic everywhere. Citizens anticipated the arrival of the virus but were otherwise helpless to mitigate its impact. Cases began to appear in the first week of October 1918, and on the 18th the Owen Sound *Sun* reported that the disease was 'Claiming More Victims Than the Battle Fronts of Europe.' There were already 800 reported cases in the town. The board of health had closed all public gathering places – schools, churches, and theatres – and the town's teachers had been recruited (on a voluntary basis) to nurse the sick who could not be accommodated in the hospital, whose beds were reserved for the severest cases. To make matters worse, food, especially farm produce, and hard coal for domestic and institutional consumption were in short supply, adding to the mounting medical crisis.[18] By the time the epidemic had run its course, about 45 days, Owen Sound had recorded more than 2000 cases representing 15–20 per cent of the population. Twenty-one deaths – a rate of 10/1000 cases – mostly of young adults, were directly attributed to the epidemic.

That there was not a greater loss of life was credited to the town's medical professionals and volunteers and, not least of all, to the G&M. 'If many Owen Sounders did not realize what the Hospital meant to the town,' the editor of the *Sun-Times* concluded, 'they have surely had their eyes opened to its value.'[19] In fact, the townspeople and their rural neighbours had not needed this latest demonstration that the G&M was essential to their well-being. After incurring operating deficits in virtually every month of 1917, the board of trustees had taken a calculated risk in the spring of 1918 and launched a one-week public fund-raising campaign under the direction of Roland Paterson, who would become the first mayor of the soon-to-be-incorporated City of Owen Sound. The objective of the campaign was to wipe out both the hospital's pre-war construction debt and its accumulated wartime operating deficits, and to provide a cushion against future inflation-induced deficits. The campaign involved a house-to-house canvass of every residence in Owen Sound, petitions to the town and county councils, and appeals to businesses. Judge Widdifield, the president of the board, explained to the public that the G&M deserved their support because it provided a better therapeutic environment than home for all but the very rich; and since the hospital wanted the patronage of the wealthy too, it also had to meet their standards, which were enjoyed, in the G&M, principally by the middle classes and the poor. The campaign was phenomenally successful, raising $15,600 in less than a month, enough to leave the board completely free of debt.[20] When a small group of private patrons provided the funding a year later for an annex to house a new laundry, ice-house, morgue, boiler room, sterilizing room, and sleeping quarters for the domestic help, the physical plant envisaged in 1909 was essentially complete, and the whole operation was, at least for the moment, financially viable.[21]

In sum, the General and Marine emerged from its wartime experience in far better circumstances than those that had prevailed in 1914. No doubt those improved circumstances were at least partly attributable to the hospital's demonstrated value in times of medical crisis such as the influenza epidemic. More generally, as a wider range of individuals representing all social classes, both sexes, and every age group gained first-hand experience of institutional medical treatment after 1910, and especially after 1914 when medical professionals were in short supply, the reputation of hospitals everywhere, including the G&M, gained added value in the public's estimation.[22] Local evidence in support of this conclusion includes the upsurge in obstetric and surgical admissions to the G&M between 1914 and 1919 (see Figure 2), the unrelenting demand for private and semi-private accommodations throughout the war,[23] and the popularity, at war's end, of the hospital as an object of voluntarism. In just one year (1918) membership in the Ladies' Auxiliary increased nearly 250 per cent as women, 'freed from patriotic charitable work,' identified the hospital as the most deserving object of their energies.[24]

No doubt some of this enthusiasm for the hospital on the part of patients and boosters alike was generated by the G&M's acquisition in December 1918 of the very last word in medical technology, an x-ray machine. The diagnostic properties of x-rays were discovered by Roentgen in 1895, and within a year were the principal subject of popular science. By 1900 x-rays were widely employed (though not in Owen Sound) by private physicians as both diagnostic tools and therapeutic devices, but hospitals were slow to acquire them, perhaps because of the expense involved and the unavailability of trained roentgenologists (the forerunners of radiologists).[25] The medical staff of the G&M had coveted an x-ray machine since before the war and in April 1914 had subscribed $550 towards its purchase, which they promoted as a sound business investment for the G&M. (Hospitals customarily ran x-ray departments on a profit-sharing basis with the physician-operator.)[26] The first x-ray machine in Owen Sound was installed, however, neither by a physician nor by the hospital but by John James, a local photographer. 'Johnny' James operated the service out of his studio during 1917–18 until the hospital board agreed to purchase his equipment and a new fluoroscope and contracted with James to operate and service the installation in the G&M. This arrangement continued until 1922, when the board was persuaded to sponsor a local physician, Dr E.E. Evans, for special training in x-ray therapy and to purchase more powerful equipment. Thereafter, the G&M's x-ray department was operated on a profit-sharing basis and became a perennial source of income for the hospital once patients overcame their initial resistance to this mysterious and intimidating process.[27] As the editor of the *Sun-Times* explained, he looked forward to the day when 'the lay mind' could grasp this 'inexplicable demonstration of the lack of solidity of matter' which seemed to prove that 'flesh and blood are subject to laws of which the race is so far completely ignorant,' but in the meantime he was thankful that this 'miracle' of x-ray therapy had come to the city.[28]

The creation of an x-ray department was merely the first step in a determined campaign planned by the medical staff to keep the G&M abreast of post-war developments in hospital care. The medical staff in 1922 – Doctors Brewster, Burt, Dow, A.L. Danard, Frizzell, Gaviller, Howey, MacDonald, Rutherford, Murray, Middlebro, and Evans – had changed little in two decades. MacDonald and Evans were the newcomers. The senior physicians and surgeons, Middlebro, Frizzell, Murray, Burt, Rutherford, Danard, Howey, and Dow, had begun their medical careers in the late 1890s as general practitioners. Typically, Frizzell, Burt, and Danard were farm boys, sons of local pioneers, and Middlebro was the son of an English stonemason who was one of the first residents of Owen Sound. They had all excelled in high school at a time when high school attendance was uncommon among farm and working-class children.

Moreover, Frizzell, Danard, Middlebro, and Rutherford all had to interrupt their education to teach public school in order to complete their medical studies. Like Dow and Howey they also interrupted their developing practices between 1900 and 1912 to pursue post-graduate specialization in surgery (Middlebro, Dow, Frizzell), obstetrics (Howey), internal medicine (Danard), pediatrics (Rutherford), and otorhinolaryngology (Burt) at highly respected British, European, or Canadian teaching hospitals during the first era of medical professionalism and specialization in Canada.[29] (Middlebro eventually was nominated FRCS and FACS). Interestingly, all of them except Howey, Murray, Evans, and Dow were graduates of the University of Toronto's Faculty of Medicine[30] and therefore learned their craft in a setting where the linkages between the theoretical and clinical aspects of medical teaching and research were particularly strong and where the modern symbiosis between physicians and hospitals first developed in Canada.[31] These were the men who in 1904 had first promoted the G&M as a centre for the scientific treatment of disease through advanced surgical techniques, and who had pushed for hospital modernization in 1909. At the end of the war they had created the Owen Sound Medical Society as a professional fraternity, as the vehicle for the continuing medical education of Owen Sound's doctors, and as a lobby to promote desirable medical initiatives in the community. As remote as they were from a major medical library, the members researched, presented, and discussed papers on current medical issues, occasionally calling in a visiting expert from the University of Toronto when their own resourcefulness failed or flagged. The society also defended its members' collective interests against 'irregular' competitors such as the city's chiropractors, and in' opposition to the determination of some local industrialists to lure doctors into 'contract' practices (unlimited medical services for firm's employees in return for an annual stipend).[32] The society, in short, was a local symbol and manifestation of the rapid evolution of medical professionalization in Canada after 1900.

The extent to which the G&M had become a 'doctors'' hospital by the 1920s is exemplified by the medical society's interest in the 'standardization' movement. Whether the hospital was a socially acceptable and financially viable institution was left to other interests to determine. Whether the G&M conformed to objectively defined minimum international standards of medical efficiency and respectability was a different matter. In 1921 the American College of Surgeons launched a hospital accreditation program. The college's objective was to define a minimum level of institutional efficiency as the standard to be met by all hospitals in which its members practised their art. Hospitals which, on inspection, met those criteria could be designated as a 'standard hospital.' The required standards included a radiology department supervised by a resident radiologist, a laboratory supervised by a qualified pathologist, a resident anesthetist, written pre-operative diagnoses and post-operative reviews for each surgical procedure performed, complete written clinical records for every patient, and a formally structured medical staff required to hold monthly meetings and to review collectively all hospital deaths.[33]

The implementation of a radiology unit at the G&M had been a first step towards acquiring the requisite facilities of a standard hospital. The medical society next persuaded the hospital board to join in a campaign to convince city council to provide a grant in partial support of a branch laboratory of the Provincial Board of Health to serve the local public health unit, the hospital, and private physicians. The physicians supported the implementation of laboratory services in Owen Sound as a necessary adjunct of physicians' private practices and of the important work of the local board of health. It had begun, after the war, to focus on a worrisome incidence of venereal disease in the city, on the health of mothers and their children through a child welfare clinic initiated by Dr Rutherford, and a school visitation program (that led, among other things, to the widespread administration of doses of iodine disguised in chocolate to combat the propensity of young girls in Owen Sound to develop goitres).[34] Agreement on the need for and financing of the lab was reached quickly, and by the end of 1921 the lab was in operation. The hospital soon became its principal client.

In the meantime the society's members discussed among themselves and with the board the implementation of the other requirements associated with making the G&M a standard hospital. Early in 1922 the society and the board jointly applied for accreditation and, following a successful site visit by agents of the ACS during the summer, the G&M was designated as a standardized hospital.³⁵ With the addition in 1923 of a motorized ambulance, the implementation in 1924 of routine lab tests for every patient admitted, and the appointment in 1925 of its own resident pathologist, the G&M had achieved, according to its promoters at least, a status superior to that of a mere 'standard hospital.' It was 'high class,' and a fitting object of civic pride.³⁶

The General and Marine Hospital was essential to the city's image of itself in the 1920s. It was a city now much changed from the rough-and-ready frontier port in which the G&M had come into existence. Between 1900 and 1910 the town's population had continued to grow apace, increasing by almost 50 per cent to roughly 12,500. With the removal of the CPR fleet, grain elevators, and depot to Port McNichol between 1912 and 1914, the decline of westward migration, and the inevitable decrease in war-related economic activity, Owen Sound was no longer an expanding community, but a city struggling to retain its population. At the same time, Grey County had experienced an era of massive rural outmigration. Its population decreased by 25 per cent in the years between 1912 and 1919.³⁷ Increasingly the city focused its attention, with some success, on attracting industrial development and improving its position as the commercial hub and market centre of Grey and Bruce counties. Following a period of post-war recession which produced widespread local unemployment in 1920 and 1921, Owen Sound's economic base began to improve modestly. A new million-bushel-capacity grain elevator, a knitting mill, and the expansion of existing businesses and industries contributed to the city's economic renewal between 1922 and 1927. By 1923 there was already a severe shortage of affordable accommodation for working men's families, many of them rural-urban migrants.³⁸ Among other things, it was the need to attract industry to provide jobs for the city's growing workforce that led to a vigorous public health campaign in the 1920s in order to promote Owen Sound as a healthy community. One result was a renewed attack on the city's longest-standing public health problem, its water supply, which was finally identified in

1926 as the source of the community's repetitive typhoid epidemics and was subsequently chlorinated.[39] But the key to a healthy community was the presence of a modern hospital. Now that good roads and instant telephone communication had eliminated the problem of distance from markets and suppliers, and cheap electrical power had eliminated high energy costs everywhere in Ontario, the president of the Ontario Hospital Association noted in 1928, the '[d]ecentralization of industry [was] on the horizon' moving away from 'crowded cities' towards 'beautiful and healthful surroundings,' and the OMA's member institutions in Ontario's outlying towns and cities should be prepared.[40]

By 1926 it was evident to patients, doctors, board members, and concerned citizens that in spite of the demonstrable quality of the services that the G&M provided, the hospital would be unable to accommodate increased demand for those services. Current usage – more than 70 per cent of annual capacity (see Table 5) – again taxed the hospital's physical resources, while the workload generated by near-capacity bed occupancy in the surgical and maternity wards in particular had strained the hospital's human resources, especially the nursing staff, beyond reasonable limits, even for a staff of historically overworked student nurses.

Although nursing as a career for women had made significant gains in the first two decades of the century in terms of public approbation of and respect for the skill and authority that the professional nurse wielded as 'the physician's hand,' it was not in the crowded wards of hospitals that the superior care provided by graduate nurses was experienced by most patients. Graduate nurses disdained hospital work except as superintendents, supervisors, or instructors, preferring instead the role of private duty nurses providing after-care for physicians' discharged patients.[41] Moreover, there is considerable evidence that, even before the war, many of the best Canadian graduate nurses were being attracted to large American metropolitan hospitals for post-graduate training and to fill supervisory positions. As one of them explained, too many American nurses were being drawn from the 'domestic servant class' because the 'New York idea of women's work' – real estate, stockbroking, theatrical booking agencies, social work, and 'the wild chase to business, to clothes and to luxuries' – had destroyed the spirit of Florence Nightingale in middle-class American women.[42] Young Canadian women, on the other hand, seemed still to be imbued with the spirit of professional altruism, and that, in combination with their apprenticeships in Canadian hospitals like the General and Marine, made them ideal nurses.

At the G&M, that apprenticeship system for student nurses changed little between 1905 and 1924. The vast majority of the training school's students, sometimes as many as 80 per cent, came from the villages and farmsteads of rural Grey and Bruce counties. (Owen Sound girls presumably were attracted by similar programs in still larger centres such as Toronto, London, or Montreal.) By 1920 the students' allowances had improved marginally, their program of instruction had been expanded to encompass a wider range of subjects, and the 1911 addition to the hospital had provided better living accommodations – four to a room and improved toilet facilities – than student nurses enjoyed in other small Ontario hospitals, where they frequently slept two to a bed.[43] But student nurses still had virtually complete charge of the wards day and night, working 12-hour shifts and taking their classes and completing their assignments during their off-duty hours. There was no time for recreational pursuits or to attend to personal matters in this gruelling regime that seemed to value stamina more than scientific accomplishment. For this reason, perhaps, the *Sun-Times* praised the G&M's graduates as a 'fine (may we say manly) type of womanhood.'[44]

After 1920 the nurses' work and domestic environment began to deteriorate rapidly as the demand for hospital beds escalated. In 1921, in order to create four new private patient rooms and one additional public ward, half the nurses were moved out of the hospital and back into the old house that had been the nurses' residence before 1912. The remainder were rehoused four to a room on the third floor of the hospital. (To avoid being housed six in a room they gave up their private study/recreation room.) Consequently the operating-room became the unofficial sanctuary of off-duty nurses.[45] This was a far cry from the separate, modern nurses' residence desired by successive lady superintendents since 1910 and strenuously recommended by every provincial inspector after 1919. '[A] city as large and as progressive as Owen Sound,' the inspector noted in 1922, should have been able to provide nurses whose 'hours are long ... and work ... exacting' with this 'necessary part of the hospital service.'[46] Moreover, inadequate and insufficient accommodation restricted the number of students who could be admitted, thereby increasing the workload of successful applicants. A further complication arose after the introduction in 1922 of the Ontario Nurse Registration Act, which created a new branch of the Department of Health to regulate and inspect training schools. In addition to designing a standard curriculum and establishing an examining board to administer common province-wide examinations for provincial registration, the Division of Nurse Registration instructed training schools to raise their admission standards and to provide instruction as part of, rather than in addition to, student nurses' duty shifts, which were restricted to a total of 58 hours per week.[47] The combined effect of these developments, including a shortage of graduate nurses and rapidly expanding admissions, was to leave the G&M with a labour crisis by mid-decade. In 1926 the hospital's nurses were reported to be generally 'in poor health' as the result of being 'overtaxed.'[48]

The growing preference among patients and their doctors for the hospitalization of the sick and the hospitals' demonstrable success in accommodating this cultural transformation were only partly responsible for the overloading of hospital facilities. Among other factors, the requirement of the 1912 Hospitals and Charitable Institutions Act that publicly funded hospitals accept tubercular and other infectious patients had the effect of turning the G&M's medical ward virtually into an isolation ward by 1922. The hospital neither wanted, nor acknowledged that it routinely admitted, tuberculosis cases, and the board threw its support behind an initiative launched by the Imperial Order Daughters of the Empire to establish a separate isolation hospital in Owen Sound, an initiative that finally failed in 1926. In the meantime the board was forced to rent a house to contain the overflow of infectious, mainly tubercular, patients.[49] The congestion in the medical ward was no greater, however, than it was in the obstetric and surgical wards. By mid-decade, when nearly half the live births occurring annually in Owen Sound were hospital births, maternity patients once again had to be housed on the surgical ward, and by December 1927 recovering surgical and medical cases 'who could be safely moved' and who no longer required intensive care were being farmed out to private homes.[50] The final straw was yet another epidemic of influenza in December 1928 which 'taxed [the hospital] to the limit' over the Christmas season and forced it to close its door to everyone but staff, patients, and the immediate relatives of terminally ill patients.[51]

By this time the G&M's board of trustees had already moved to mitigate the problems associated with a 55 per cent increase in admissions between 1919 and 1928 and an increase in bed utilization from less than 50 per cent of the hospital's capacity in 1914 to more than 70 per cent in 1928 (see Table 5). In 1926 the board began to debate the necessity of building a major addition to the hospital. The projected cost, $50,000, was a major deterrent until two private benefactors (both board members), D.M. Butchart and John Harrison, offered to subscribe $10,000 each. With these gifts in hand, the hospital's board decided to sponsor a referendum in January 1927, asking the citizens of Owen Sound to be similarly generous in approving a by-law to add three quarters of a mill to the local rates in order to provide the hospital with $6000 annually for its capital and maintenance requirements. In the meantime the board and the Ladies' Auxiliary were required to forgo their usual fund-raising activities, only to have the proposed by-law declared illegal by the provincial government, which would only permit the hospital corporation, as a charitable trust, to receive a capital grant from the city.[52] Consequently, a year of fund-raising was lost while the board went back to the ratepayers in January 1928 with a new by-law to permit the city to issue debentures in order to raise $50,000 for hospital construction. The by-law was approved, tenders were opened in April, and in June ground was broken by Muntz Construction of Toronto, low bidder at $67,000.[53]

Sir William Mulock, chief justice of the Supreme Court of Ontario, officially opened the new wing on 17 July 1929, although it was not ready to receive patients until the autumn. By then the costs of constructing and furnishing the addition had ballooned to $94,000.

The board, free of debt for nearly a decade, was faced with the prospect of raising a further $21,000 to retire a new mortgage, and with a deficit on the year's operations as the result of higher maintenance costs arising principally from the need to employ more graduate nurses to cope with the hospital's workload.[54] There was nevertheless ample cause for celebration. The new addition was heralded as a 'substantial, enduring ... thoroughly modern ... monument of the zeal of the hospital board,' the 'fulfillment of ... a dream of the local medical staff,' and 'the acme of efficiency for the care and treatment of the sick.'[55]

*The Canadian Hospital*, the new (since 1924) voice of hospital professionalism in Canada, carried a major feature on the G&M's addition in its October 1929 issue. The article recalls a familiar interior landscape. '[P]ale expanses of wall space' in the wards contrasted with the deep red tones of the cushioned battleship linoleum that ran through gleaming off-white corridors. Spacious terrazzo-tiled bathrooms (with hot and cold running water) on each floor (and in every private room) made housekeeping easy. From their beds with adjustable springs and legs, the latest word in hospital furnishings, patients could summon nurses with a 'silent call' button. Each floor's diet kitchen, complete with steam table and a refrigerator, was serviced by dumb-waiter from the main kitchen. The basement contained a lecture hall and a demonstration room for the school of nursing, and a nurses' common room. Enlarged administrative space was provided, as well as an improved doctors' room and a larger x-ray department. All of the hospital's service lines were accessible through a false ceiling, a major innovation, and the entire building was fireproof. Most important of all, the addition housed two state-of-the-art operating-rooms, a separate anesthesia room, and the best sterilizing equipment that money could buy.[56]

The addition provided space for 45 patients in 17 private rooms, 4 semi-private wards (2 beds each), and 4 public wards (5 beds per ward). But the net gain was only 36 beds because there had not been sufficient funds, once again, to provide a separate nurses' residence, and 4 private rooms and the female public ward in the 1893 wing had to be reclaimed for nurses' accommodations. The nurses were promised that a residence was the next item on the board's agenda, and the local citizens were assured that they would never again 'be refused admission for lack of accommodation.'[57]

Once again, the community's needs had been met by a collaborative effort on the part of public officials, private benefactors, ordinary citizens, local organizations, and hospital volunteers. Private patrons provided $20,000 in major financing, the city's debentures another $50,000. Subscriptions from ordinary citizens accounted for another $10,000, while the Ladies' Auxiliary contributed nearly $3000. Local service and charitable organizations, fraternal lodges, and businesses furnished and decorated the private wards and supplied the sterilizing equipment. The main operating-room was a private commemorative gift. The editors of *The Canadian Hospital* habitually castigated hospital administrators and trustees for failing to sustain the support and sympathy of the public for the costly revolution that had transformed hospitals from 'boarding homes' for the sick poor into 'highly scientific institutions for the treatment, study and prevention of disease.' Only in smaller communities, they thought, had the spirit of voluntarism and the 'personal element that should exist between the public and the hospital' survived the transformation.[58] They might have been referring to Owen Sound and Grey County.

The principal evidence for a developing estrangement of the public from the hospitals was a growing consumer revolt in the United States against the high cost of hospital care. By the late 1920s this disaffection had spread to Ontario, led, according to knowledgeable commentators, by 'the great middle class of self-respecting people of moderate means'[59] who were seeking neither the free treatment available to the poor nor the first-class care available to the rich. 'What they want, and what is needed, is a hospital where medical skill would be adequate, the accommodation comfortable and the patient would not be haunted with the spectre of "the cost." '[60] According to the Dominion Bureau of Statistics, average hospital charges had increased 90 per cent between 1913 and 1928 and were escalating at a rate of roughly 2 per cent per year. During the same period public ward charges had increased 92 per cent, semi-private ward rates 82 per cent, and private ward rates 96 per cent.⁶¹ Hospitals frankly acknowledged that the rates they charged their paying patients were increasing faster than public ward charges. They blamed government for its failure to pay the full cost of maintaining indigent patients, leaving hospitals with shortfalls in operating income, which had to be recovered from paying patients. These patients then faced the prospect of financial ruin as the result of hospitalization, unless they were willing to accept the stigma of being hospitalized on the free list.⁶² As Table 6 illustrates, both the proportion of patient-days subsidized by the government and provincial funding as a percentage of hospital incomes in Ontario had been declining steadily since the turn of the century. The slight, but important, reversal of these trends in the mid-1920s is evidence of what the hospitals feared most, an increase in the numbers of indigents seeking free care at the expense of paying patients or, even worse, evidence that hospital costs were pauperizing formerly paying patients. It was to become a recurring theme in the public and political debates over hospital financing that unfolded in Ontario over the next 30 years.

For the moment relations between the General and Marine Hospital and the community remained free from these recriminations. One reason was the active involvement of an especially experienced group of trustees in the management of the hospital. The citizens who attended the official opening of the new wing in July 1928 were told that they owed their new hospital largely to the efforts of the board's president, Joseph R. McLinden.⁶³ The manager of the city's Public Utilities Commission, McLinden was Owen Sound's Thomas Edison. At the age of 19, apparently without formal training, he supervised the construction of the hydroelectric dam and machinery that harnessed the power of Inglis Falls for S.J. Parker's electric illumination company, later the Owen Sound PUC. In 1928 McLinden was serving his eighth term as president of the trust having served previously for four years as chairman of the board's Property Committee. McLinden was not merely an able administrator. He was, evidently, very aware of the pace and the content of the health care revolution and was determined to keep the G&M abreast of those developments as far as its resources would allow.⁶⁴ Serving with him in 1927–8 as vice-presidents or chairmen of the

TABLE 6
Admissions, patient stays, income, and expenditures, Ontario public general hospitals, 1880–1950

| | 1880* | 1885 | 1890 | 1895 | 1900 | 1905 | 1910 | 1915 | 1920 | 1925 | 1930 | 1936 | 1941 | 1946 |
|---|---|---|---|---|---|---|---|---|---|---|---|---|---|---|
| No. of patients admitted | 5,302 | 6,617 | 9,094 | 16,161 | 29,572 | 37,736 | 52,321 | 83,161 | 130,459 | 152,198 | 215,623 | 218,133 | 254,598 | 408,551 |
| Admissions per M pop. | 2.8 | 3.3 | 4.3 | 7.6 | 13.6 | 16.3 | 20.9 | 30.9 | 45.1 | 48.6 | 63.8 | 60.4 | 60.4 | 75.1 |
| Average stay (days) | 35 | 34 | 30 | 28 | 24 | 20 | 20 | 18 | 15 | 14 | 14 | 15 | 14 | 12 |
| Av. cost per patient day ($) | 0.57 | 0.63 | 0.71 | 0.72 | 0.76 | 1.09 | 1.30 | 1.55 | 2.84 | 3.40 | 3.65 | 3.06 | 3.47 | 5.03 |
| Av. income per patient day ($) | 0.66 | 0.72 | 0.82 | 0.95 | 0.81 | 1.08 | 1.25 | 1.64 | 2.82 | 3.35 | 3.97 | 3.46 | 3.84 | 5.58 |
| Sources of annual income (%): | | | | | | | | | | | | | | |
| Municipalities | 25.5 | 22.9 | 25.4 | 17.1 | 16.2 | 18.4 | 20.1 | 29.9 | 17.6 | 16.7 | 14.9 | 24.4 | 16.3 | 10.5 |
| Province | 18.3 | 12.7 | 10.6 | 7.8 | 6.3 | 9.2 | 10.6 | 7.8 | 6.0 | 9.2 | 8.2 | 10.9 | 6.3 | 4.7 |
| Subscriptions/gifts | 15.8 | 15.5 | 16.5 | 30.2 | 26.4 | 15.5 | 13.4 | 8.1 | 9.5 | 7.6 | 6.7 | 4.8 | 4.9 | 5.1 |
| Investments/interest | 10.4 | 8.9 | 8.6 | 3.8 | 3.6 | 4.8 | 4.2 | 3.3 | 2.1 | 2.2 | 2.2 | 2.1 | 2.9 | 2.2 |
| Patients' fees | 9.0 | 16.8 | 18.1 | 19.3 | 35.3 | 48.6 | 51.7 | 50.8 | 64.8 | 64.3 | 68.0 | 57.8 | 69.6 | 77.5 |
| Proportion of patient days subsidized by the province (%) | 84.8 | 85.9 | 90.7 | 81.9 | 79.3 | 69.6 | 63.5 | 61.1 | 44.7 | 57.3 | 51.7 | 63.4 | 37.2 | 10.5 |
| Patients' fees as % of maintenance costs | 10.4 | 18.9 | 20.8 | 25.0 | 37.7 | 47.7 | 49.6 | 53.9 | 64.2 | 63.0 | 74.0 | 65.2 | 77.1 | 86.0 |

*Data for years up to 1939 are for 12 months preceding 30 September of year noted.
SOURCES: Province of Ontario, Legislative Assembly, Sessional Papers, Annual Reports of Returns to Inspector of Prisons and Charities and Department of Health, 1880–1946

board's property, finance, and house committees were a group of men – R.D. Little, Alfred Creasor, John Parker, and Dr George Holmes – who had amassed a total of 44 years of service on the board. Little was one of the city's largest retail grocers, Creasor the local police magistrate, Parker the treasurer of Grey County, and Holmes the county registrar of deeds. If to these names are added the next longest serving executive members of the board between the first (1910) and second phases of hospital expansion – the entrepreneur D.M. Butchart, the lumbermen F.W. and E.J. Harrison, and Mrs Elias Lemon, wife of the city's most successful wholesale grocer – these nine trustees (including McLinden) exercised the executive functions of the board for 84 (70 per cent) of the 120 person-years represented by those responsibilities in these two crucial decades of the G&M's history. Later this historical continuity of leadership would be criticized, and eventually restricted, as a barrier to popular participation in the management of the city's most important secular charity (see Chapter 4). In the meantime, although medical philanthropy was by no means limited to a narrowly defined group of benefactors, the task of ensuring that the G&M operated efficiently and economically from day to day had become the special preserve of a small, dedicated cadre of volunteers representing a large reserve of managerial and financial expertise, and a long history of familial involvement in the affairs of the hospital.

The G&M's progress was also due to the ministrations of a succession of extremely able lady superintendents – Margaret Redmond, Ethel Woods, Jennie McArthur, Georgina Thompson, and Maude Stirling – who since 1913 had kept costs within reasonable limits without sacrificing the quality of hospital services. Just how difficult their task was can be surmised from a comparison of Tables 5 and 6. While average maintenance costs per patient day increased nearly 30 per cent in Ontario's public general hospitals between 1919 and 1930, the G&M's costs of necessity remained relatively constant because the G&M's income per patient-day increased at only half the rate (20 per cent) of the provincial average. The G&M's administrators, in short, worked close to the margin, which was largely defined by annual income from patient fees. These accounted for a much greater proportion of the G&M's annual income than was the case generally among the province's hospitals. The fees charged to paying patients in effect underwrote a significantly greater share of the G&M's costs of maintaining all patients than was the case in other hospitals. During periods of relative prosperity hospital management under these conditions was tolerable. Conversely, any major social or economic dislocation that might make hospitalization less accessible to paying patients threatened the relatively secure foundation on which the G&M rested in 1929.

As Table 7 indicates, by 1926 the medical reasons for admitting patients to the G&M represented a remarkably modern pattern in comparison to the earlier history of hospital morbidity in the G&M and are quite similar to post–Second World War trends throughout Ontario. Together, respiratory disease, diseases of the digestive system, pregnancies, genito-urinary ailments, and accidental injuries – acute illnesses which required direct medical intervention including, in more than half of these admissions, surgical intervention – accounted for the majority of admissions to the G&M in the 1920s. In addition, by 1929 the x-ray department was processing 700 cases a year, including nearly 400 fractures and about 50 candidates for 'deep therapy' treatments of, among other things, malignancies, exophthalmic goitre, and enlarged glands. The radiologist, Dr Gordon Webb, had even acquired a portable unit for home treatments.[65] The G&M may still have lacked many of the amenities, services, and specializations of larger or wealthier metropolitan institutions; but it was no less capable of healing the sick according to the latest tenets of medical science and within the limits of current therapeutic effectiveness, which flowed from a mix of radical science, clinical trial and error, and still a good deal of the traditional 'holistic' medicine practised by physicians who were just a generation removed from the era of the country doctor.[66]

Between 1918 and 1930 the General and Marine Hospital enjoyed unprecedented popular support, not only as an indispensable agency of individual well-being, but as a monument to the city's ambition to be, and to be seen as, a progressive community with all of the amenities of modern society. In spite of the rapidly rising costs of individual and family health care that now marked the G&M as a business rather than a charity, the hospital was the single

TABLE 7
Comparative frequency (%) of admissions/discharges by diagnostic categories, Ontario hospitals, 1900-47

| Category | Owen Sound G&M Hospital | | Ontario general hospitals | |
| --- | --- | --- | --- | --- |
| | 1900 | 1926 | 1938 | 1947 |
| Infective and parasitic | 29.8 | 4.5 | 2.3 | 1.5 |
| Neoplasms | 3.1 | 3.9 | 4.7 | 4.6 |
| Allergic, endocrine, etc. | 0.0 | 1.4 | 2.8 | 2.1 |
| Diseases of blood & blood-forming organs | 0.0 | 0.2 | 0.5 | 0.4 |
| Mental, psychoneurotic | 6.5 | 0.9 | 0.6 | 0.1 |
| Diseases of nervous system & sensory organs | 0.8 | 3.2 | 4.0 | 2.8 |
| Diseases of circulatory system | 3.4 | 2.6 | 2.9 | 5.4 |
| Diseases of respiratory system | 8.8 | 20.2 | 4.6 | 18.3 |
| Diseases of digestive system | 17.2 | 13.1 | 26.4 | 12.6 |
| Diseases of genito-urinary system | 9.5 | 6.7 | 6.8 | 6.1 |
| Delivery, complications of pregnancy, puerperium | 3.1* | 12.0* | 16.6 | 27.2 |
| Diseases of skin/cellular tissue | 0.0 | 0.3 | 1.8 | 2.8 |
| Diseases of bones & organs of movement | 4.2 | 1.4 | 1.2 | 1.5 |
| Congenital malformations | 0.0 | 0.0 | 0.4 | 0.2 |
| Diseases of early infancy | 0.0 | 0.1 | 12.4† | 0.3 |
| Symptoms, senility | 0.0 | 0.1 | 0.1 | 3.0 |
| Special admissions | 4.2 | 0.6 | 0.9 | 0.9 |
| Accidents/poison/violence | 6.5 | 7.1 | 8.2 | 8.3 |
| Not stated | 2.3 | 11.1 | 2.6 | 0.7 |
| Live births | 0.8 | 10.6 | | |

*Excludes births
†Includes births
SOURCES: G&M Hospital, admissions register, 1900-1, 1925-6; Province of Ontario, Department of Health, Division of Medical Statistics, *Survey of Public General Hospitals in Ontario*, Part IV (Toronto 1940), Table X, p. 20; Province of Ontario, Department of Health, *Report of the Health Survey Committee*, Volume I (Toronto 1950) Table A54, p. 91

most important object of voluntary public generosity in the county, a secular charity sustained by all classes in the community as a matter of collective self-interest. For the moment at least, the hospital's publicity could legitimately claim that anyone who was 'once a patient' was 'always a booster' of the G&M's growing sophistication as a workshop for the efficient and economical production of scientifically generated good health.

# 4
# 'Sickness Is an Expensive Luxury': Depression, War, and the Crisis of Health Care, 1930-49

In retrospect, of course, the timing of the decision to undertake a major expansion of the Owen Sound General and Marine Hospital as an expression of faith in the city's industrial future was less than ideal. Within three months of the inauguration of full service in the G&M's new facilities in October 1929, the first local economic casualties of the developing world-wide depression had become a visible social and political problem. By the winter of 1933-4, at the peak of unemployment in Owen Sound and the deepest trough of depression nationally, 2000 people – roughly 17 per cent of the city's population – were dependent on direct public relief. Their situation improved only marginally until business and agriculture in Grey County, as in the rest of Ontario, returned to something like 'almost normal' conditions in 1937.[1] In the meantime these indigents shared with the 15-20 per cent of their countrymen who also found themselves living on welfare the 'shabby and humiliating sort of half life ... feared and hated by most Canadians ... and yet increasingly accepted as the only real alternative to starvation ...' and homelessness.[2]

Food, clothing, and shelter were not the only necessities of life required by these victims of the Depression. Sickness, always a threat to the financial security of working men and their families in good times, became an even graver hazard with the onset of widespread economic hardship. Moreover, evidence collected by the Ontario Department of Health in the late 1930s suggests that as poverty became more widespread it was accompanied, as might be expected, by an increase in illness, especially health problems associated with poor nutrition, bad living conditions, the psychological strains of poverty and dependence, and complications arising from reluctance to seek or accept medical relief. The number of chronically ill elderly persons increased as well.[3] Who was to provide medical relief for the once-again swelling ranks of the sick poor, and who would pay? From the perspective of Ontario's public general hospitals, the stigma of the Victorian poor-house that they had deliberately shed between 1890 and 1920 now threatened to reattach itself to, and to undermine, their new enterprise, which they energetically defended as an industry selling a scientifically produced commodity – health – to those who could afford its justifiably rising price. Caring for larger numbers of patients, rich or poor, was not the problem. Recovering the full cost of treating every patient, however, had become the well-established measure of hospitals' progress from charitable institutions to efficient businesses. The question of who would pay for the rising tide of indigent patients, and how much, was therefore of vital economic and political concern to hospital professionals and lay trustees alike.

In fact, the hospitals had rehearsed publicly all of their arguments on this subject before the Depression struck. Between 1921 and 1925 the proportion of patient-stay days subsidized by the provincial government began to increase after declining continuously from 1880 until the end of the war. This increase in the number of indigent patient-days was not accompanied, however, by a similar expansion of provincial or municipal liability, in spite of the hospitals' rapidly escalating operating costs. By the mid-1920s the recently formed Ontario Hospital Association had embarked on a major campaign to convince the government to improve provincial and municipal subsidies for public ward patients, preferably up to the full cost of their maintenance. The OHA estimated that in 1926 the cost to its member institutions of treating indigents was $1.3 million more than the hospitals' statutorily defined income for these purposes. The cost of providing this subsidy had been passed on to paying patients in the form of higher user fees, said the association, whereas the income generated by higher subsidies would have allowed the hospitals to treat paying patients at cost and to use some of that income to improve hospital services for all patients. The problem, the OHA's president told the government in 1927, was that the idea of the hospital as a dispenser of welfare was as obsolete as the title of the department (Prisons and Charities) to which hospitals reported. Medical philanthropy was no longer the only mandate, or even the most significant aspect of the work of the modern hospital; but it demonstrably had become the chief hindrance to the determination of a fair price, for the paying consumer 'of moderate means,' for a product to which 'legitimate business principles should ... be applied.... The hospital has [a] very necessary service to render ... and the recipient must pay.'[4]

The Canadian Medical Association, after flirting with the idea of state-supported medicine earlier in the decade,[5] now supported the hospitals' position on the question of medical charity. 'I am convinced that we have gone about far enough in the direction of free treatment,' the president of the CMA announced in 1927. The 'Robin Hood' principle of 'supertaxing' the 'provident' middle class to provide health care for the 'non-provident' sick poor was 'inadequate for the distribution of scientific medical care' in the twentieth century. Hospitals 'half filled with people who cannot, or will not, or do not pay' deprived those institutions of the income necessary to become 'dispenser[s] of medical science' through 'the efficiency of specialism' and the 'team-work' of the 'specially-equipped centre' which bore the same relationship to modern health care, the CMA pointed out, that the factory did to the industrial revolution.[6] A private physician put the matter rather more succinctly. Hospitals which were accessible only to the recipients of charity were inaccessible to doctors except as providers of charity. Hospitals had to be maintained as 'the agents through which the latest achievements of science are made available ... by the profession' to physicians' paying private patients.[7]

This campaign brought only a limited, immediate response from the provincial government, which finally agreed in 1928 to raise the municipal indigent rate from $1.50 per day to $1.75 and its own grant for public ward patients from 50 to 60 cents per day.[8] The combined grants represented perhaps two-thirds of the hospitals' reported average cost of maintaining one public ward patient for one day in 1928. Nevertheless, the hospitals had reason to hope that a government-appointed Royal Commission on Public Welfare would give greater consideration to their concerns; but when the Ross Commission reported in 1930, it provided little solace for them. The commissioners concluded that hospital accounting practices were so diverse as to make it virtually impossible to discern the actual effects of indigent admissions on hospital costs and revenues across the system. The commission pointed out that hospitals in some communities were genuinely hard pressed while others were relatively well off, and argued that this was clearly a reflection of local priorities. Their *Report* consequently recommended that community-defined standards of hospital care sustained by community-generated grants appropriate for achieving those standards for all classes of the local population represented a better mechanism for ensuring social justice than provincial subsidization of the full costs of medical relief.[9] As if to re-inforce the commission's perception, in 1931 the government repealed the 1912 Hospital and Charitable Institutions Act and replaced it with a new Public Hospitals Act which spelled out a far more rigorous set of municipal responsibilities for the provision of medical relief to indigents. At the same time, the government reminded hospitals that they were 'primarily charitable institutions ... [where] ... [t]he latest discoveries and developments in equipment for diagnosis and treatment, as well as the most advanced medical and surgical skill, are at the disposal of the suffering poor for the asking.' The question of who pays was irrelevant. The real problem was that hospitals were simply inept in the management of their revenues.[10] There the matter stood until the Depression and its related crisis in health care had run their course.

In Owen Sound, the city council was not unduly alarmed by the signs of spreading unemployment during the winter of 1929-30. The city had experienced high rates of seasonal unemployment in the past, and apart from appointing a relief officer and establishing a registry of men looking for work, no further action was taken. Even as late as October 1930, when the employment registry had swelled to 250 (mostly laid-off factory workers), a council deputation sent to Toronto to discuss the government's plans for providing unemployment relief returned convinced that Owen Sound's problems were not as serious as those faced by other communities.[11] By Christmas, however, demand on the city's benevolence fund was running at $400 a week, half of it for medical relief, and the *Daily Sun-Times* noted that there were now families facing 'actual suffering and want.'[12] The situation worsened during the winter of 1931 and the return of spring brought no respite. In the first six months of 1931 the city spent $16,000 on direct relief, and a number of public works projects – sewer and gas main expansion, roadwork, and public beautification projects – provided employment for only 125 of the more than 400 men seeking work.[13] The onset of winter was expected to bring with it an even larger number of men and families requiring public welfare. Most of them, said the editor of the *Daily Sun-Times*, were 'people who have never before been in need of assistance and who hesitated to ask for it'; but their exceptional circumstances now demanded co-ordinated and concerted action among all of the city's official and volunteer social service agencies 'to see that no family or person received more than they are entitled to or need, and that the needs of those who are actually without means and require assistance received such help.'[14] Council responded to this growing crisis by creating a welfare board to co-ordinate and control all forms of relief, including medical charity.

The effects of the Depression on the operations of the General and Marine Hospital were not immediate. Although the recently expanded hospital treated 50 fewer inpatients between October 1929 and September 1930 than it had in the previous 12 months (see Table 8), annual fluctuations of this magnitude were normal. Moreover, three-fifths of the patients admitted during the year requested accommodation in the hospital's now higher-priced private and semi-private wards, with the result that income from patient fees increased nearly 14 per cent and at year's end there was a modest operating surplus. The board assumed that the G&M was now 'largely self-financing' and began planning for the incorporation of laboratory services in the hospital.[15] But even as the trustees were congratulating themselves on the success of their expansion

TABLE 8
Summary data, G&M Hospital, 1930–9

| | 1930–1 | 1931–2 | 1932–3 | 1933–4 | 1934–5 | 1935–6 | 1936–7 | 1937–8 | 1938–9 |
|---|---|---|---|---|---|---|---|---|---|
| No. of patients treated | 1,232 | 1,033 | 1,246 | 1,399 | 1,621 | 1,691 | 1,758 | 1,471 | 1,596 |
| Average stay (days) | 14 | 15 | 13 | 12 | 11 | 11 | 11 | 11 | 10 |
| Income/patient day ($) | 2.35 | 3.57 | 3.38 | 3.08 | 3.21 | 3.26 | 3.36 | 3.68 | 4.02 |
| Cost/patient day ($) | 3.57 | 2.93 | 3.27 | 2.63 | 3.36 | 3.48 | 3.65 | 4.33 | 4.03 |
| Occupancy rate (%) | 34.9 | 40.0 | 43.3 | 48.3 | 49.6 | 49.3 | 50.1 | | |
| Av. no. of patients/day | 34 | 39 | 42 | 44 | 49 | 48 | 48 | 45 | 54 |
| No. of beds | 95 | 96 | | 81 | | 80 | 80 | | |
| No. of medical admissions | 385 | 316 | 304 | 316 | 374 | 397 | 442 | 517 | |
| (%) | 31.3 | 30.6 | 24.4 | 22.6 | 23.1 | 23.5 | 25.1 | 35.1 | |
| No. of surgical admissions | 550 | 587 | 608 | 674 | 831 | 875 | 845 | 779 | 947 |
| (%) | 44.6 | 56.8 | 48.8 | 48.2 | 51.3 | 51.7 | 48.1 | 53.0 | 59.3 |
| No. of obstetric admissions | 148 | 130 | 149 | 188 | 183 | 209 | 210 | 229 | |
| (%) | 12.0 | 12.6 | 12.0 | 13.4 | 11.3 | 12.4 | 11.9 | 15.6 | |
| No. of births | 149 | 132 | 147 | 188 | 187 | 210 | 212 | 235 | 235 |
| Total income ($) | 51,540.54 | 50,973.19 | 51,663.85 | 50,042.31 | 57,996.73 | 57,738.64 | 55,527.68 | 61,017.64 | 78,730.43 |
| Total patient fees ($) | 41,144.78 | 35,032.11 | 34,991.87 | 36,757.95 | 42,335.95 | 43,127.41 | 49,105.59 | 49,197.19 | 59,677.57 |
| No. of x-ray patients | | | | 983 | | | 1,480 | | 1,780 |
| Value of x-ray work ($) | | | | | | 6,590.50 | 8,722.90 | 10,306.53 | 12,932.20 |
| Value of lab work ($) | | | | | | | | | 2,061.50 |
| Annual surplus/deficit ($) | | | –10,000.00 | | | –4,790.10 | –8,817.30 | –13,130.00 | –249.96 |
| No. of salaried nurses | 4 | 4 | | 4 | 4 | 6 | 8 | 6 | |
| No. of pupil nurses | 28 | 28 | | 36 | 36 | 41 | 43 | 32 | |
| No. of private beds | 60 | 58 | | 48 | | 47 | 51 | | |
| No. of public beds | 38 | 38 | | 33 | | 33 | 29 | | |

SOURCES: G&M Annual Reports; Board of Trustees Minutes; Owen Sound *Daily Sun-Times*; Province of Ontario, Legislative Assembly, Sessional Papers

program, the medical society was meeting to discuss ways of dealing, both as private physicians and as hospital staff doctors, with the growing number of patients seeking medical charity at the surgery door. Their concern was echoed, in a different way, by a spate of newspaper articles anticipating the need for either a government-sponsored scheme of medical insurance or the creation of 'government commandeered and salaried physicians' who would treat patients 'regardless of their ability to pay.'[16]

What the doctors anticipated, and what in fact transpired over the next three years, was the emergence of a double-edged problem for the city's health care providers. Among the sick who could still afford to pay for treatment, there was a growing preference for home care by their private physician or treatment in his surgery as an alternative to more costly hospitalization. The sick poor, on the other hand, sought medical charity from the hospital and from any physician willing to render aid under any conditions. As physicians became increasingly overburdened with medical relief work, to the detriment of their private practices, they turned to the welfare board and to the hospital's public wards as solutions to their problem. The evidence (Table 8) for this conclusion includes, among other things, the history of admissions to the G&M after 1930 (and the consequent effect on the hospital's financial stability). As the Depression deepened locally, the number of paying patients – more particularly those who normally would have occupied private wards – swiftly declined. The average duration of hospital stays declined as well, and the G&M's overall occupancy rate plummeted. The result was that in the hospital's 1931–2 fiscal year income from patients' fees was one-third less than it had been in 1929–30. But total hospital income had decreased by just 18 per cent because municipal payments for indigent patients had risen 66 per cent. By 1935 the largest category of admissions to the G&M consisted of patients with unstated or undefined illnesses, evidence of the custodial character of their hospitalization and the philanthropic reasons for their admission. The hospital nevertheless experienced operating deficits, more than $10,000 in 1932, the inevitable result of the displacement from the hospital of paying patients who had once sought preferential care by a growing population of welfare patients. President McLinden voiced the opinion of hospital trustees throughout Ontario in expressing the hope that 'the time will come when the man with a meagre ... income will not have to pay hospital expenses with money that should be used to support his family in frugal comfort.'[17] Many Owen Sounders had already made that decision, however reluctantly, and more would as time passed. Patient fee income continued to decline until 1934 and did not return to pre-Depression levels until 1937. Annual operating deficits grew larger and accumulated so that the hospital's operating losses, by 1938, amounted to more than $13,000 (see Table 8). The board could only institute such economies as were consistent with the continued efficient operation of the hospital and wait out the circumstances that had caused the G&M to revert to its original identity as a charitable institution providing basic care to predominantly public ward patients, many of them referred to the hospital by the town's overworked doctors.

It is impossible to know with any certainty what percentage of the hospital's patients were welfare cases requiring wholly subsidized care. However, the board calculated that the cost of treating indigents in 1933 was $7200.[18] Assuming that these patients stayed on average 13 days at the board's reported average cost of $3.27 per day, the sum represents the care of 170 patients – at least 15 per cent of all admissions and probably closer to 20 per cent on the further assumption that the cost was calculated at the lower statutory rate for indigent care. Whatever their number, in 1933 these cases represented just the tip of a social policy iceberg, responsibility for medical relief, which had become a significant problem in Owen Sound. Physicians could no longer cope with the demand for medical charity and were having difficulty sustaining their schedule of fees for paying patients, many of whom were living on reduced incomes. The doctors hoped to persuade the city to appoint paid medical relief officers and to pay 50 per cent of the doctors' normal fees for the welfare cases they had treated so far. The G&M's board insisted that the city council pay the full cost of caring for indigent patients because the hospital's falling income, now largely derived from its public ward charges which were pegged, below cost, by legislation, no longer covered the hospital's operating expenses. For its part, the finance committee of city council was reeling under the staggering costs of welfare for 1775 men, women, and children in 1933 and was determined to control, as far as possible, its liability for medical relief. Consequently, the welfare board was instructed to appoint two medical relief officers (and later a third) under supervision of the medical health officer. For a salary of $75 per month they were to provide medical care, including prescription drugs, to patients approved by the welfare board. At the same time, the G&M was informed that except in life-and-death emergencies it was not to admit local indigents unless they were accompanied by a signed order from the mayor's office. Doctors received a similar injunction against admitting welfare patients, especially maternity cases, to hospital without the approval of one of the relief doctors and a mayor's warrant; and they were to refrain, as members of the hospital's medical staff, from ordering expensive tests and drugs for indigents except when absolutely necessary. The purpose of these orders was to restrict the treatment of welfare recipients to home care provided by the relief doctors as a means of keeping the lid on the most costly component of the city's welfare commitments.[19] Ironically, and as if to prove the point Ontario's hospitals had been making for nearly a decade, controlling the flow of indigents to the hospital proved to be the first step in improving the G&M's annual balance sheets. The second, far more difficult to achieve, was to recover the $12,900 in unpaid accounts that accumulated between 1930 and 1935.[20]

In the midst of these difficulties, three further problems, largely unrelated to the exceptional social circumstances of the Depression, intruded on the hospital's operations. The first was, at least on the surface, a management problem in the x-ray department. The radiologist, Dr Webb, had been reprimanded by the board in February 1932 for his 'slovenly appearance' (according to testimony later presented in court) and for smoking in the presence of patients. The problem persisted and in April an ad hoc committee of the board and the medical staff met to discuss the problems of the radiology department, which may or may not have included some confusion over the board's policy regarding responsibility for collecting accounts in the department. Matters did not improve. In mid-July Dr Webb was given six weeks' notice of his dismissal effective 1 September, and the department was padlocked pending the appointment of a replacement.²¹ Claiming that the hospital's rules were 'an insult to any self-respecting practitioner,' and that he was the victim of a much larger conspiracy, Webb subsequently sued the board for wrongful dismissal and was awarded $420 and costs, because the defence had been unable to prove conclusively that Webb had wilfully disobeyed or disregarded direct orders from the president of the board.²²

There the matter might have ended. But in the meantime Webb had returned to private practice, announcing his radiographical services in newspaper advertisements which offered a money-back guarantee if he failed to cure goitre, skin diseases, tonsillitis, and glandular disorders painlessly without unnecessary operations. The Ontario College of Physicians and Surgeons was alerted and began an investigation which ended in hearings before the college's discipline committee and its council. Webb was asked to refrain from advertising his money-back guaranteed 'cure,' refused to comply, and was struck from the college's register. On appeal, in June 1934 the Supreme Court of Ontario upheld the college's decision to bar Webb for 'infamous and disgraceful conduct.'²³

To the disruption and uncertainty caused by the Webb affair was added, in the summer of 1932, an ominous threat from the provincial committee on nurses' training to withdraw its approval from the G&M's training program. The decision appears to have been based on (admittedly well-founded) rumours about the student nurses' living conditions, rather than on reports of actual inspections, since the board was able to appeal successfully for a site visit before a final decision was taken. The trustees acknowledged that there was a problem, but argued that the G&M, as the only 'standard' hospital in a very large area, was an essential nurses' training facility.²⁴ The fact is that the need for a proper separate nurses' residence had been evident since at least 1904, and that the students in particular had been moved around and in and out of the hospital whenever the need for additional treatment beds had arisen. By 1932 some of them were housed in the original (1893) wing of the hospital, the rest in an old house the board occasionally resurrected for these purposes.

It was primarily the hospital accommodation for the nurses, and to a lesser extent the quality of their training program, that exercised the inspector of nurse training schools when she visited the G&M in June 1933. The students' accommodations were 'shabby and unattractive,' poorly furnished, and overcrowded. The assistant superintendent was too preoccupied with her duties as obstetrics supervisor to fulfil her role as the students' principal instructor in nursing practice. And the student nurses had too frequent contact with tubercular patients.[25] One solution was to employ more graduate nurses and fewer students, the substance of a specific request to the board from a joint committee of the national and provincial nursing associations who hoped to make work for unemployed graduate nurses by persuading hospitals to reduce admissions to their nurses' training schools. But the G&M relied more than ever on its training school to keep its wage bill in check[26] and was determined to retain the school's accreditation.

The Ladies' Auxiliary (renamed the Women's Hospital Aid in November 1933) stepped into the breach to forestall further negative assessments of the training school. They persuaded the welfare board to conscript relief recipients to provide the necessary labour, and they put up the funding to refurbish the 1893 wing completely as a nurses' residence. When the inspector returned 10 months later, she congratulated the board on the 'general transformation' that had taken place and on its specific accomplishment of 'providing comfortable and homelike surroundings for the graduate and pupil staff.'[27] Less tractable were the problems subsequently identified by the inspectorate: providing for an expanded curriculum and additional graduate staff to supervise it, and raising admissions standards. A full-time nursing instructor, graduate supervisors for each floor, and formal affiliation with larger hospitals where the students could be sent for training in dietetics, sanatorium nursing, and pediatrics were regarded by the inspectorate as minimum criteria for a sound curriculum. The G&M achieved the latter objective by affiliating with the Detroit Children's Hospital and the Ontario

Hospital in London, where student nurses (at their own expense) served brief internships. Requiring all applicants for admission to the school to have matriculated proved unrealistic relative to the hospital's labour requirements, and expanding the graduate staff was economically impracticable. Nevertheless, by 1937 the inspectorate was satisfied that Owen Sound was an ideal place, both geographically and in terms of the quality of its program, for a nurse training school.[28]

The final administrative crisis of the Depression era involved Bertha Hall, who was appointed lady superintendent in October 1930.[29] Throughout the worst years of the Depression, Superintendent Hall had won repeated accolades from the board, the press, the nursing inspectorate, and the medical staff for her efficient management of the hospital under difficult, sometimes impossible, circumstances. In the spring of 1936, however, the board was informed by the medical staff that every department in the hospital was 'seething with disloyalty' because relations between the graduate nursing staff and Miss Hall had become 'intolerable.' The board met four times to review these reports. The third meeting ended in an especially rancorous debate followed by a vote called to decide Miss Hall's fate. Members voted nine to five in favour of retaining Miss Hall's services and the president promptly resigned. Six weeks later the question was reopened; board members reversed their earlier vote, and the president was asked to resume his chair. It seems clear, however, that after 15 consecutive terms as president, Joe McLinden had at last found an issue that would relieve him of a burden he had been trying to shed, unsuccessfully, for at least three years. His successor, Dr G.W. Holmes, was left to resolve the matter, which came to a head in December when the dietitian and four graduate ward supervisors submitted their resignations, citing as their reason 'lack of co-operation' on the part of the lady superintendent. Finally, in spite of their belief that Miss Hall was 'largely responsible for the present excellent financial and physical position of the institution,' board members sided with the medical staff and the ward supervisors. Miss Hall was allowed to resign 'of her own free will' and was given three months' salary in return.[30]

Amidst this half-decade of turmoil the work of the hospital

progressed slowly. There were some essential developments, largely as the result of the generosity of private benefactors. The G&M at last acquired 'iceless refrigeration' in 1932 and an integrated fire-alarm system in 1935. In 1933 the aging Wappler x-ray unit was replaced by a more powerful Westinghouse machine, one of whose attractions was that it did not interfere with local radio reception. The new radiologist, Dr Gordon French, proved to be both a competent technician and an astute business man, and thereafter the department was a major source of income for the hospital. Dr A.L. Danard, one of the hospital's longest-serving physicians, provided the hospital with a modern nursery in 1936 to improve the 'scientific routine' of infant care, and in May 1937 the hospital appointed its first laboratory technician and medical records librarian.[31] But after five years of depression-induced economies, these improvements and innovations, however essential, scarcely scratched the surface of the hospital's requirements, beginning with the need to pay off its mortgaged $20,000 debt for its 1929 expansion, to replace aging, outmoded, and worn-out equipment, and above all to get out from under an accumulated operating deficit incurred as the result of the dislocation of the hospital's normal admissions profile. With business returning to more normal patterns after 1936 – the G&M again operated at 50 per cent of capacity, revenues returned to pre-Depression levels, lengths of stay increased, as did the demand for private accommodation in 1937 (see Table 8) – the board decided that the time was ripe to launch a new appeal for civic and public support.

The decision opened a pandora's box of sometimes bitter and always heated debate about the General and Marine Hospital's role in the community. It began innocently enough with a request to the city council from the G&M's board for a grant of $4000–5000 to launch a public fund-raising campaign. The board's case was built on the argument that the hospital had operated throughout the Depression with no civic assistance and, moreover, had treated the municipality's indigent patients at a fraction of the real cost of their maintenance. A $5000 grant actually represented less money, the board argued, than council might have spent if it had given the G&M annual grants throughout the Depression or paid full fare for its hospitalized welfare cases. This line of reasoning won the support of most councillors, but others were less easily convinced. Among the minority there was a strongly held opinion that the Owen Sound Medical Society, which was still negotiating with council in the hope of recovering fees for services to indigents during the Depression, should contribute to the G&M's operating revenues in the form of a levy on each physician of at least $500 for hospital privileges. In the end the majority opinion prevailed, and a grant of $4000 was endorsed.[32] But the matter did not end there.

Five months later, in March 1939, the hospital board was back at city council seeking a further grant of $8000 as the first instalment of the $200,000 the trustees thought they could profitably spend on the hospital. Citing a 'half-hearted' autumn fund-raising campaign as an example of the board's inability to manage its own affairs adequately, the chairman of the city's finance committee returned to an earlier theme: 'the doctors want to build up the hospital as a medical centre; it is their workshop' over which neither council nor ordinary citizens had any control. Consequently, it was argued, the hospital was managed in the interests of a minority and persisted in offering services that it was financially unable to support. The committee returned to the idea that physicians should pay for the privilege of treating their private patients in the G&M.[33]

The suspicion that hospitals increasingly served the interests of doctors rather than patients was one of the by-products of the professionalization of medicine and of hospital modernization in the first quarter of the twentieth century. It was a growing source of tension within hospitals as well as between medical professionals and the public, and was exacerbated by the circumstances of the Depression. In Owen Sound, these charges elicited a lengthy public response from the board's president, Dr Holmes, who challenged councillors to justify 'their very erroneous impressions' of an institution that pumped $60,000 a year into the local economy, derived 75 per cent of its income from patient fees, treated the city's indigent population at a price far below cost, and was managed voluntarily by lay trustees on behalf of the hospital's real owners, the citizens of Owen Sound. Council, he said, could choose to starve the hospital into mediocrity or, worse, force the board to drive up the rates for paying patients and make hospital services even more inaccessible; or, council could acknowledge that the G&M was at least as important as the library, the new hockey arena, or the city band, and make a modest contribution to help restore its physical plant and its fiscal stability.[34] Six months later council agreed to a grant of $4000.

As the editor of the *Daily Sun-Times* astutely remarked, however, whether the city gave the G&M $4000 or not was really beside the point. The point at issue, in the aftermath of the Depression, was who should pay for health care. What the council should be doing, in his opinion, was devising a contributory hospital insurance scheme for the citizens of Owen Sound. 'It has been said that there are two classes only that can afford to be sick – those who have money for doctors and hospital bills and those who have no money and have to be treated at the expense of the municipality ... [In] the average "in between" family sickness is an expensive luxury.'[35] In fact, such a scheme – Associated Medical Services, Incorporated – had already been launched, and Owen Sound's physicians were even then seeking information about it. Moreover, city council took the newspaper's advice and debated 'the hospitalization burden,' concluding that the city might have to broaden its support of hospitalization to include 'borderline' cases of patients who were neither indigents nor wholly self-supporting citizens.[36]

Health care, and more particularly hospital, economics was the subject of much public debate by the time the Depression had run its course. Privately sponsored group hospitalization insurance was one answer to the growing problem of accessibility to health care services and, especially, the burgeoning cost of hospitalization and hospital maintenance. Throughout the Depression academics, civil servants, and vested interest groups had examined the problems of modern health care from every conceivable perspective. As early as 1932 the federal government's Commission on Social Insurance had been provided with an exhaustive report demonstrating the feasibility of a national contributory health insurance program that would provide a minimum standard of accessibility and care for every Canadian in return for premiums that even families with very modest incomes could afford.[37] Similarly, by 1939 the Ontario Hospital Association had begun to investigate a non-profit hospitalization insurance plan which it proposed to offer through its member institutions.[38] Even the Canadian Medical Association became a supporter, during the Depression, of hospital insurance. Ontario's Ministry of Health undertook an extensive survey between 1936 and 1940 of trends in hospitalization in the province in an attempt to identify the source of the health care crisis and to recommend ways to resolve it. The survey yielded three quite separate explanations for the increased demand for hospital services. The first two had nothing to do with the unusual circumstances of the Depression. In the first place, the survey concluded, the hospital had simply become, since 1900, the primary health care centre for the vast majority of the population, and for certain acute medical problems – digestive disorders, childbirth, accidental injuries, and diseases of early infancy (pre-natal and neo-natal) – had become almost indispensable. Second, the province had an aging population that generated higher case frequencies and longer stays in hospital, which tended to increase demand for services, tie up beds, and therefore increase hospitals' costs. To this already heavy traffic, the Depression had added large numbers of indigent patients who, relative to their actual numbers, accounted for a disproportionate share of stay days and a disproportionate claim, in the form of maintenance costs, on hospital income from all sources in relation to the much lower income these indigent patients generated for hospitals. Coupled with the determination of middle-class patients to avoid hospitalization at all costs as their incomes declined, the effect on hospital revenues was critical. The report concluded that the return to normal social and economic conditions would largely remove indigent patients as a factor in hospital economics, and with them the problem of accessibility and rising costs to paying patients resulting from their presence.[39]

The ministry's consultants might have used the General and Marine Hospital as a case study. As the data in Table 9 suggest, during the Depression patterns of hospital morbidity changed dramatically. In both 1930–1 and 1935–6 the proportion of patients admitted with unspecified or undetermined maladies represented the largest single category of admissions. Undoubtedly many of these were welfare or chronically ill elderly patients whose attending

TABLE 9
Patterns of hospital morbidity, selected diseases, G&M Hospital, 1930–40 (percentages)

| Year | 1930–1 | 1935–6 | 1941 |
|---|---|---|---|
| Nervous/sensory system | 5 | 3 | 6 |
| Respiratory disease | 17 | 19 | 17 |
| Digestive system | 12 | 11 | 13 |
| Genito-urinary | 5 | 7 | 8 |
| Pregnancy/puerperium | 15 | 15 | 24 |
| Accidental injury | 8 | 2 | 10 |
| Not stated | 30 | 37 | 4 |
| Total | 92 | 94 | 82 |

SOURCE: G&M admissions registers, 1930, 1935, 1941

physician determined (assuming that there was an alternative) that hospital care was preferable to home care. On the other hand, the proportion of patients admitted with serious injuries declined as unemployment spread, just as the proportion of maternity cases declined as the city implemented its policy of forcing indigent mothers to undergo home childbirth. Finally, the seven major causes of hospitalization during the Depression constituted a much larger percentage of all admissions than they did after 1940 when the range of ailments for which people were prepared to be hospitalized (or which physicians were prepared to document) expanded. These observations can be correlated with the information in Table 8, which suggests that the effects of the Depression dampened hospital usage only briefly (1930–3) and hardly affected the flow of surgical admissions. Yet occupancy rates remained low, the duration of patients' stays grew shorter, income declined, and deficits accumulated.

It seems that in Owen Sound, as in the rest of Ontario, the flight of the paying patient from the hospital (especially from its private wards) except in dire emergencies, the tendency towards shorter and therefore less costly stays, the development of other forms of medical relief for indigents, and the use of the hospital's services for the custodial care of certain welfare patients all contributed to the creation of a hospital system that could no longer afford to treat the sick poor without larger infusions of public funds or greater profits from the care of paying patients who had learned that they could not afford the cost of medical care on those terms except at their peril. The crisis had been brewing since before the First World War. As the Second World War approached, whether these problems would resolve themselves with the return of better times, as the Ontario government's experts thought, or whether their resolution would require a major reassessment of Canadian social policy, was already decided in the mind of Prime Minister Mackenzie King.

For the time being, however, Canada, in 1939-40, had to soldier on, and the G&M had to adjust quickly to wartime conditions on the home front. Local civil defence planning was premised, at least initially, on the possibility of the air war spreading to North America, and the G&M aimed at 'peak efficiency' in order to be ready for any emergency. But efficiency was difficult to achieve amid the conditions imposed by the war. For example, the hospital was unable to attract a class of qualified student nurses in either March or September 1940 because of better employment opportunities for women generated by the war.[40] Similarly, the appeal of 'dramatic stories' of the assistance required 'in faraway places' was blamed for a sudden decline in subscriptions and donations 'to provide for the needs of our civilian population who are doing a truly good job in the homeland.'[41] By 1943 half of the G&M's medical staff had enlisted in the medical corps leaving not only the hospital, but the city as well, short of qualified physicians. Worse, perhaps, a shortage of graduate nurses developed as training school underenrolments, enlistments, and a bidding war among hospitals for the services of RN's took their toll on smaller communities like Owen Sound.[42] But even if nurses had been available the G&M could not have housed them. The old nurses' residence (the converted house) was commandeered until 1942 as a military hospital for a Polish regiment training in the county, the converted 1893 wing of the hospital only housed part of the nursing staff, and the demand for patient beds had strained available space to the limit.[43]

In May 1941 admissions to the G&M achieved a historical high of 219. The hospital treated on average 79 patients a day, one short of capacity. The record remained unbroken until September 1946,[44] but in the interim, as Table 10 indicates, the G&M had annual occupancy rates in excess of 70 per cent and minimum average daily patient loads of 70. Over all, annual admissions increased 89 per cent during the war years, but surgical admissions increased 122 per cent and hospital births 150 per cent. The flow of patients through the x-ray department kept pace with the rate of admissions (suggesting that every patient was routinely x-rayed). Evidently more than just health care delayed by the Depression was responsible for this unabating upsurge in hospital business. The return to full employment, the advent of contributory group medical insurance, the appearance towards war's end of such 'wonder' drugs as streptomycin and penicillin, and the revival, after a long hiatus, of the public's preference for hospital-centred health care undoubtedly were all factors contributing to this unparalleled growth in hospitalization. A specific factor, illustrated by the increase in the number of hospital births, was women's growing preference not only for hospital-based obstetrical care, but for painless childbirth. One result, apparently, was an increase in the G&M's infant mortality rate, which the medical society carefully monitored and attributed to the craze for 'streamlined' labour in which induction and sedation rendered childbirth 'free from discomfort and recollection' but took its toll in the form of 'dead or damaged babies.' The physicians resolved to limit their intervention to assisting nature, 'the master surgeon.'[45]

The General and Marine Hospital failed, however, to benefit from this resurgence of demand for hospital care. Although the hospital's total annual revenues increased between 1940 and 1945 by 119 per cent, its annual bill for wages, supplies, and services climbed by 160 per cent, and its total annual costs for maintaining patients escalated 148 per cent. By 1945 patients' fees accounted for nearly 90 per cent of the hospital's annual income and contributed more than 90 per cent of the costs of patient maintenance (see Table 10). The hospital had become a business dependent for its success on selling its life-giving products to paying consumers. It was not a successful venture by the usual standards of free enterprise. Deficits accumulated (more than $20,000 by 1945), the physical plant and its equipment deteriorated, and the trustees began to doubt their ability to sustain the hospital's central role in the life of the city.[46]

TABLE 10
Summary data, G&M Hospital, 1940-5

| | 1940 | 1941 | 1942 | 1943 | 1944 | 1945 | 1946 | 1947 | 1948 | 1949 |
|---|---|---|---|---|---|---|---|---|---|---|
| No. of patients treated | 1,938 | 2,155 | 2,470 | 2,683 | 3,271 | 3,484 | | 4,244 | 3,178 | 3,457 |
| Average stay (days) | 11 | 11 | 11 | | 10 | 9 | | | 9 | 9 |
| Income/patient day ($) | 3.79 | 3.95 | 4.62 | 4.70 | 5.31 | 6.17 | | | | 9.80 |
| Cost/patient day ($) | 3.81 | 3.95 | 4.39 | 4.19 | 4.93 | 5.76 | | | | |
| Occupancy rate (%) | | 79.4 | 76.7 | 74.1 | | 82.8 | | | | |
| Av. no. of patients/day | 60 | 64 | 70 | 78 | 79 | | | | | 101 |
| No. of beds | | 80 | 92 | 92 | | 95 | 95 | 101 | | 103 |
| No. of medical admissions (%) | | | | | | | | | | |
| No. of surgical admissions | 946 | 1,035 | 1,171 | 1,223 | 1,779 | 2,106 | | | 2,147 | 2,242 |
| (%) | 48.8 | 45.0 | 47.4 | 45.6 | 54.4 | 60.4 | | | 67.6 | 64.9 |
| No. of obstetric admissions (%) | | | | | | | | | | |
| No. of births | 274 | 352 | 406 | 470 | 515 | 488 | 635 | 828 | 692 | 667 |
| Total income ($) | 80,896.84 | 92,392.50 | 118,911.00 | 117,065.13 | 150,766.14 | 177,093.28 | | | | |
| Total patient fees ($) | 70,716.47 | 84,024.45 | 93,965.31 | 100,956.90 | 135,905.93 | 157,938.62 | | | | |
| No. of x-ray patients | 2,445 | 2,456 | 2,833 | 3,112 | 3,176 | 3,610 | 4,407 | 4,763 | 4,553 | 4,928 |
| Value of x-ray work ($) | 14,531.75 | 15,322.50 | | | | | | 25,162.82 | | |
| Value of lab work ($) | 4,767.00 | | | | | 6,982.00 | | | | 10,744.00 |
| Annual surplus/deficit ($) | -643.04 | | | | -8,308.60 | -7,702.00 | 7,436.00 | -35,000.00 | -27,000.00 | -43,321.00 |
| No. of salaried nurses | 6 | 23 | 20 | 34 | | 42 | 34 | 38 | 37 | 34 |
| No. of pupil nurses | 43 | 47 | 30 | 30 | | 24 | 26 | 30 | 26 | 30 |
| No. of private beds | | 51 | 59 | 59 | | 62 | 62 | 64 | | 64 |
| No. of public beds | | 29 | 33 | 33 | | 33 | 33 | 37 | | 39 |

SOURCES: G&M Annual Reports; Board of Trustees Minutes; Owen Sound *Daily Sun Times*; Province of Ontario, Legislative Assembly, Sessional Papers

In the aftermath of the Depression, the board had concluded that it would have to work at re-establishing popular sympathy for the hospital as an object of charity. Toward that end the trustees created a public relations committee in 1943, an idea first mooted by hospital professionals in the late 1930s to counter patients' charges that hospitals were too business-like and government's opinion that they were too wasteful and inefficient.[47] The committee had its work cut out for it. The hospital, according to its annual report for 1944, was in 'very grave financial condition' as the result of its accumulated deficit and its urgent need to improve its plant and equipment. Yet another municipal grant of at least $5000 to forestall a major fee increase and to initiate yet another public appeal for funds was required. But city council had been advised that the G&M's deficits were merely the product of creative accounting: if the donations of private benefactors were calculated as operating income and if the hospital's claimed depreciation on its buildings and equipment was excluded from its operating costs, the G&M was earning a healthy profit. The board protested that the charges were unfair, but the damage had been done. Several benefactors cancelled their ongoing commitments, and the council responded with a grant of only $3500. In desperation the board turned to the good offices of Mayor Garfield Case (who attained national notoriety 10 months later when he defeated General A.G.L. MacNaughton, Mackenzie King's hand-picked candidate, in a federal by-election), who arranged an interview with the minister of health, R.P. Vivian. The minister informed the G&M's deputation that the government had no intention of burdening municipalities with additional statutory responsibilities for hospitals. He suggested, however, that the board was free to negotiate an arrangement with the City of Owen Sound whereby the General and Marine Hospital would become a civic hospital owned and operated by the city.[48]

By the end of 1944 the board was grasping at straws when it received a lengthy communication from a retired trustee, C.A. Eberle, reflecting on the hospital's problems. Eberle concluded that the organization of the board and its relationship to both the hospital and the community were the sources of many of its difficulties. Too many board members, he suggested, were identified with vested interests and had served those interests for too long. The board needed constant infusions of 'new blood' to deal with the managerial, financial, public, political, and professional relations of a modern hospital and required a leaner structure of more active subcommittees. Similarly, the operations of the hospital required a new administrative structure to replace the outmoded office of lady superintendent and to reflect the institutional complexities of a modern health care centre.[49]

The board tackled these proposals in three stages during 1945 and 1946. First it reformed itself, re-emerging as a board of governors with a new committee structure consisting of executive, management, finance, and public relations committees. Next, it proposed changes in the trust's by-laws to limit executive office-holding on the board to no more than three consecutive years, to establish an attendance criterion for continuing membership on the board, and to make every citizen who attended the annual meeting a voting member of the trust. These changes were approved in February 1946 during one of the most well-attended (200 people) and most enthusiastic annual meetings since 1920. The new board interpreted this as a signal that the hospital's fortunes were changing.[50] It remained only for the 'new blood' to devise a better administrative structure for the G&M, and to test the waters of public approval of the now 'truly representative' board.[51]

The proposed administrative changes were developed in 1946 and introduced in 1947. Reta Brown, the superintendent, became the superintendent of nursing with responsibility for the training school and the nursing staff. James Clark, who had served as administrative secretary for five years, became the hospital's administrator supervising the non-medical staff and overseeing all of the hospital's operations. Together, Brown and Clark constituted the G&M's executive officers reporting directly to the management committee to which the medical staff, now reorganized into obstetrical, surgical, medical, pediatric, outpatient, physiotherapy, and radiology services, also reported directly.[52] This administrative restructuring effectively brought to an end an anachronistic Victorian system of hospital management that survived in many smaller hospitals well into the twentieth century. In fact, the day had long passed when a lady superintendent, trained professionally as a nurse, but assumed, by virtue of her sex, practical experience, and the custodial function of a hospital, to be an ideal domestic housekeeper, authority figure, accountant, and business manager, could effectively co-ordinate all of the operations of a sizeable hospital alone, with or without additional professional training. By the 1930s it was already widely recognized that hospital administration was itself becoming a highly specialized field of expertise to be acquired only partly through experience. Hospital journals began to carry lengthy articles on 'Training in Hospital Administration,' the first textbooks of hospital management began to appear, and by the early 1940s the first postgraduate programs in hospital adminstration became available. Indeed, the G&M's reorganization might have come straight out of Bachmeyer and Hartman's *The Hospital in Modern Society*, a widely used textbook.[53] It seems likely, however, that the horizontal separation of administrative functions at the G&M in 1947 was less a question of creating distinct spheres of professionalism than a simple recognition that the institution had become too complex for a single manager.

While this corporate restructuring was progressing, the newly elected board struck out boldly to recover lost time. It contracted with a professional fund-raiser to design and lead a campaign to go forward with a referendum seeking ratepayers' approval for a municipal grant of $300,000 for hospital expansion, and with a request to Grey County Council for a grant of $100,000. The long-range goal of the campaign was a building fund of $1 million to sustain a major expansion of the hospital. The campaign got off to an auspicious start. By early summer the citizens of Owen Sound had contributed $93,000 in voluntary subscriptions and had approved the municipal grant.[54] It remained only for the county and the province to contribute with equal generosity. When Leslie Frost, treasurer (later premier) of Ontario, proposed in his 1947 budget to provide provincial funding to hospitals for capital construction projects and to increase operating grants on the basis of total public ward capacity rather than indigent occupancy rates, the G&M's finance committee made yet another pilgrimage to Toronto. There they learned that their plan to add 51 active treatment beds, 28 chronic care beds, and 18 pediatric beds, though not the nurses' residence, should be eligible for support.[55] Since the board had at hand funds apparently adequate to build the long-overdue nurses' residence, it immediately called for tenders in the almost certain knowledge that with depression, war, and popular indifference behind it, and with an era of peace, prosperity, and provincial funding in the offing, the Owen Sound General and Marine Hospital would at last realize its much-delayed promise as a 'great organization of healing.'[56]

Their optimism was premature. Grey County Council (which had given only maintenance grants to the hospital since 1930) failed to acknowledge the board's request for funds to support its building campaign or operating deficit. The board, in retaliation, slapped a 15 per cent surcharge on the accounts of all county patients admitted to the G&M. Worse, it soon became evident that there would be no additional provincial funding in 1947 at least, either for construction programs or to help offset the rising tide of red ink in the operating accounts of Ontario's hospitals. The minister of health offered instead to lend the G&M an 'efficiency expert' and volunteered the suggestion that Grey and Bruce counties (both now served by the hospital) should contribute equally to the G&M's operating income. The last straw was the low tender for the proposed nurses' residence, $80,000 higher than the $140,000 estimate the board had used.[57] With a projected deficit of $35,000 in the offing and uncertain prospects for the augmentation of its building fund, even $140,000 seemed too much for the board to risk. It settled for a 150 by 30 foot prefabricated RCAF administrative hut purchased from the War Assets Disposal Corporation for $975.[58]

These setbacks seem incongruous at a time when even the Department of Health acknowledged publicly that hospitals like the G&M could not pay their bills, collect their accounts, or satisfy public demand for their services. Moreover, the department accepted unquestioningly, though it would not state publicly, that the General and Marine in particular was 'obsolete ... badly overcrowded, and ... lacking suitable accommodations for student nurses.'[59] But in the immediate post-war period Premier George Drew's Conservative provincial governments had neither the tax bases nor the ideological disposition to intervene directly in the medical market-place. The province of Ontario had been an especially adamant opponent of a proposed federally funded national health insurance scheme as a threat to provincial autonomy. At the other end of the political spectrum, the Conservatives regarded legislative interference in the traditional independence of voluntary social institutions such as hospitals and universities as unwarranted, even if Queen's Park had been able to relieve their financial distress.[60] As for the province's hospitals, they had been lobbying hard at least since 1925, not for massive, direct government involvement in their affairs, but only for a much more limited intervention: full payment of their actual costs of caring for indigent patients so that the paying 'patient of moderate means' could still afford hospitalization without acquiring the Victorian stigma of a public ward 'charity' case. One thing was certain. By the late 1940s patients, politicians, physicians, and philanthropists could all agree that something had to be done to resolve the social and economic problems of medical care in Ontario. It only remained to determine what was to be done.

# 5

## 'What Can a Drowning Man Afford for a Life Jacket?' The Politics of Health Care, 1949–69

The difficulties confronting the Owen Sound General and Marine Hospital in 1949 constitute a catalogue of the problems faced by public general hospitals everywhere in Ontario in the post-war era. Population growth (Owen Sound's population had increased to about 16,500 by 1951), the demand for increased accessibility to the hospital, overcrowding, higher operating costs, deteriorating or obsolete buildings and equipment, the need to provide a wider array of hospital services involving larger numbers of specially trained personnel and more sophisticated equipment, and above all the problem of identifying the extraordinary financial resources required to underwrite a second modernization of hospital care tested the perseverance of hospital administrators and governors as never before. For patients the benefits of medical science had never seemed more inestimable, with the advent of a diagnostic and pharmacological revolution, or more elusive, as hospitals attempted to resolve their problems by charging all that the traffic could bear for their services. In the end neither patients nor hospitals could afford the post-war price of medical progress, but neither could society afford the social costs of restricting accessibility to modern health care to those individuals or communities best able to compete for its services and benefits. The health care system in general, and hospitalization in particular, necessarily became a question of national and provincial social policy in the era of post-war reconstruction.

In the midst of the war, in fact, a broadly based inquiry into the problems of Canada's health care system had been undertaken as part of a sweeping assessment, initiated by the Liberal government of Prime Minister W.L.M. King, of the need for social security legislation following the massive dislocation created by the Great Depression. An advisory committee on health insurance (the Heagerty Committee) consulted widely among health care experts, providers, users, and policy-makers (including Sir William Beveridge, author of Britain's national health scheme) before preparing its report, which included draft legislation to create a national program of universal health insurance which would have provided, among other things, a full range of hospital services.[1] The proposal was welcomed, at least in principle, by the Canadian Hospital Council, whose spokesmen told the committee that hospital trustees had become completely discouraged by the controversy over who should pay for the hospitalization of indigent patients, and that their paying patients, in the meantime, had become socially handicapped by their inability to budget for unanticipated hospitalization given the constant inflation of maintenance charges made necessary by the indigent problem. What the council wanted was to preserve the autonomy of hospitals as 'democratic' philanthropic institutions within a system of hospital care made affordable to paying middle-class patients by relieving them of the need to support, with their fees, the hospitalization of those who could not pay.[2] Interestingly enough, an influential study prepared for the Commons' Special Committee on Social Security concluded that while the 'general case' for universal health insurance was the potential for increased productivity among healthier low-income Canadians, the 'special case' was the well-documented inability of the 'average wage-earner ... to provide adequate medical care for ... his family.'[3]

Wartime conditions prevented King from implementing his social security program, but in the course of the first post-war federal-provincial conference he presented his 'Green Book' proposals to the provincial premiers. One of the proposals was for a federally assisted program of provincially administered health care initiatives, including grants for health research, hospital construction, health care improvement, and health insurance.[4] The adamant opposition of Premier Duplessis of Quebec and Ontario's George Drew forestalled co-operation in these matters, however, and it was left to Ottawa to begin the process of inducing the provinces to participate, in the first instance with a program of grants for hospital construction, professional training, and health care research introduced in 1948.[5] Hospital insurance remained the province of commercial carriers such as Associated Medical Services, Inc. and non-profit insurers such as Blue Cross (sponsored co-operatively by provincial hospital associations) which had emerged in the aftermath of the Depression to offer voluntary group health insurance in response to growing public demand. By 1948 one in every four patients – one in every five paying patients – admitted to hospital in Ontario carried some form of hospitalization insurance, a statistic which the government interpreted 'largely as a response by the growing number of persons in the middle income groups' to the need for orderly budgeting for sickness in the face of the spiralling costs of hospitalization.[6] This conclusion was confirmed by the Canadian Sickness Survey undertaken by the Dominion Bureau of Statistics in 1950–1. The survey found that among the 86 per cent of all Canadian families with medical expenses, 58 per cent subscribed to some form of prepaid medical/hospital insurance plan (50 per cent carried hospitalization insurance), and that Canadians in 1950–1 spent as much on premiums for hospitalization prepayment plans as they did for direct hospital care.[7]

This scenario was being played out in Owen Sound as well. The 'appalling shortage of beds' at the G&M by 1950 was attributed by its board to both the increased availability of affordable hospitalization insurance and the growing sophistication of the hospital's diagnostic and treatment facilities.[8] Before the war, medical specialization at the G&M, with the exception of surgery, obstetrics, otolaryngology, and radiology, had been an adjunct of general practice. For example, Dr A.L. Danard, the G&M's consultant in internal medicine for 30 years, was first and foremost a respected family physician. By 1950 the medical staff included specialists in pathology, anesthesia, gynecology, and ophthalmology who, like their counterparts in the other areas of medical service, increasingly limited their activities to their fields of specialization.[9] Demand for their services had created such a crush of patients that the hospital's hallways were crowded with beds. The solution proposed by the board in 1947, a 117-bed addition, neatly coincided with the announcement of the federal government's National Health Grants program to commence in 1948, which provided matching funds for hospital construction and renovations. The Department of Health's unwillingness to approve these plans for funding in 1948 was a serious enough setback. Its continuing refusal to do so throughout 1949 and 1950 on the grounds that the G&M's plans for a 200-bed hospital were too pretentious for such a small community increased the problem of overcrowding to the point where the G&M was forced to restrict admissions and curtail elective surgery.[10]

A larger hospital, whatever its size, obviously threatened to compound the General and Marine's continuing financial problems associated with the provision of increasingly costly services to more and more patients. Many of them had to be treated 'regardless of their ability to pay,' while the hospital's income from the rest was 'governed by the ability ... to pay' fees that reflected the effects of inflation, the wartime improvement in wages for hospital employees, and the need to sustain higher staff/patient ratios to meet the paying patient's expectations of better service.[11] For example, the growth of the G&M's workforce between 1930 and 1956, as illustrated by Table 11, reflects the increasing labour-intensiveness of hospital care, the growing complexity of the hospital's operations, which required larger numbers of non-medical staff, and the continuing shortage of both graduate and student nurses during and after the war. Although the number of graduate nurses per 100 patients treated daily quadrupled between 1930 and 1941, thereafter the G&M's salaried nursing complement grew at half the rate of the lay staff, which increased 67 per cent between 1941 and 1951.[12] Many of these additions were orderlies and nurses' aides hired partly to constrain the hospital's wage bills, but primarily to alleviate the burden borne, as the result of the shortage of registered nurses everywhere, by the nursing staff who, as patient loads grew, were increasingly restricted to the care of the acutely ill.[13] The result was a quantum leap in the hospital's wage bill, which had represented just 30 per cent of total operating expenditures in 1930.

TABLE 11
G&M Hospital workforce, 1930–56

|  | 1931 | 1941 | 1951 | 1956 |
|---|---|---|---|---|
| Nurses/100 patients treated daily | 63 | 94 | 76 | 86 |
| Graduate nurses/100 patients daily | 8 | 39 | 51 | 51 |
| Student nurses/100 patients daily | 55 | 61 | 25 | 35 |
| Other employees/100 patients treated | 40 | 70 | 117 | 138 |
| Wages as % of total hospital expenditures | 30 (est.) |  | 57 | 67 |

SOURCE: Province of Ontario, Ministry of Health, Government Returns, 1930–56 (G&M copies)

By 1951 wages constituted nearly three-fifths of operating expenditures; they would soon exceed 66 per cent as the workforce continued to expand and wage settlements improved dramatically, at least partly through the intervention of newly certified bargaining units. The board had been warned in 1945 that 'the low scale of salaries and wages which [prevailed] prior to the war' was history, and that wages would be the principal source of hospital costs in the future.[14] By 1951, average wages at the G&M were increasing at the rate of 5 per cent annually, while the hospital's total wage bill was growing by about 9 per cent per year.

Meeting these wage bills and other operating expenditures – food, maintenance, laundry, supplies, drugs, heat and power, housing for nurses – which constituted the remaining 40 per cent of the G&M's budget was a matter for the new arithmetic of hospital accounting. From the hospital's inception in 1893 until the end of the Depression, charges to paying patients had consisted primarily of just three components: maintenance fees (captured in room rates), operating room surcharges (since 1907), and surcharges for x-rays (since 1922). This income was almost always less than the hospital's annual operating expenses. Government grants and private donations sometimes bridged the gap, but more often than not deficits accumulated: hence the ongoing struggle between Ontario's public general hospitals and the provincial government over its failure to pay a larger share of the cost of maintaining indigent patients in particular and public ward patients generally. The hospitals argued, without success, that hospital care would soon be inaccessible to their paying 'patients of modest means,' as hospitals increased private ward rates and piled surcharges onto their basic maintenance charges in order to offset losses incurred from treating indigents below cost (see Chapters 3 and 4).

How far that threat had become a necessity by 1951 can be seen from a breakdown of the G&M's income from paying patients which then comprised 97 per cent of the hospital's total annual revenue. Of the fees paid by patients, charges for room, board, and nursing care represented just 62 per cent. Surcharges for radiology, laboratory, operating and delivery room services, for drugs, and for medical sundries accounted for the other 38 per cent. The average patient who remained in one of the hospital's public wards for nine days paid, on average, $10.80 per day, as the hospital reported. But his bill represented only $6.60 per day ($\times$ 9 = $59.40) for maintenance and, on average, $37.00 in surcharges.[15] Of course many paying patients, given their preference for private or semi-private accommodation, paid much more. Reviewing these surcharges, the Department of National Health and Welfare conceded that this was certainly 'an easier method of helping to finance part of the growing cost of extending skilled medical care to indigent patients, than begging from hard-pressed municipalities.'[16] But these tariffs were limited by the paying patients' ability to pay, and, in Owen Sound as elsewhere, were rarely ever enough, between 1945 and 1959, to avoid an annual deficit in the hospital's accounts. Faced with continuing operating deficits, put under extreme demographic pressure to expand but unable to contemplate expansion without raising the spectre of higher costs and deepening debts, dependent on the willingness of paying patients or their insurers to pay rapidly inflating charges for the use of second-rate facilities and for care at the hands of larger numbers of unskilled staff, hospitals like the G&M, the provincial legislature was told by Dr Mackinnon Phillips (Owen Sound's MLA and soon to be minister of health) in 1950, were 'up against a stone wall.'[17]

These problems, and a number of others, were finally documented in a comprehensive provincial health survey conducted by the Ontario Department of Health from 1948 to 1950 under the National Health Grants program. The three-volume report of the Ontario Health Survey Committee noted that in post-war Ontario patient demand for care in public general hospitals like the G&M had created a shortage of nearly 10,500 acute treatment beds. Another 4600 beds were obsolete and required immediate replacement. Childbirth, diseases of the respiratory and digestive systems, accidental injuries, genito-urinary and circulatory disorders, in that order, were the leading causes of hospitalization. Owing to the efficacy of modern diagnostics, surgery, and drugs, hospital stays for these illnesses and injuries were much shorter, and hospitals therefore had been able to respond to the growing health consciousness of Ontarians by treating many more patients in existing facilities. That was no longer possible in terms of available space, the added expense of providing a wider variety of more costly, labour-intensive services to a rapidly expanding population, or the financial condition of the province's public general hospitals. The survey disclosed that in 1948, for example, nearly 11 per cent of the patients admitted to general hospitals were indigents unable to pay for their own care. They accounted for 42 per cent of the days of care provided in the general hospitals' public wards and were the principal source of hospital operating losses. This was because the provincial government's most recent (1947) revision to the statutory grants payable for indigent and public ward patients encouraged hospitals to allocate too high a proportion of their beds to subsidized patients whom the hospital had to treat below cost as the price of eligibility for essential provincial and municipal support. Consequently, indigents were maintained largely at the expense of paying patients who paid surcharges for extra services amounting to 51 per cent of their hospital bills. Hospitals, the report concluded, were not like other businesses and could not be expected to recover their costs from their clients, or to finance the expansion of hospital care out of revenues inadequate even for their daily operations. The province's 1400 voluntary lay trustees were 'responsible citizens,' but the problems of the modern general hospital were beyond their control. What Ontario required, said the committee, was a hospital commission to 'study, administer and control the operations and expansion of Ontario's hospital facilities.'[18]

About a similar suggestion from the mayor that the Owen Sound General and Marine Hospital ought to be run by a tough-minded three-man commission capable of keeping its costs under control, the editor of the *Daily Sun-Times* remarked that the 'broadly representative' G&M board was perfectly capable of 'maintain[ing] the best in hospital care, to which patients ... are entitled.'[19] Doing so in 1950, however, had become a perplexing and exasperating exercise in political manoeuvering to advance the hospital's cause on two fronts – the recovery of its operating losses, and approval for and funding of its expansion plans. The G&M's operating losses could be attributed to different sources from year to year – $41,000 in unpaid accounts in 1947, a $27,000 loss in 1948 as the result of reducing admissions by 400 to control overcrowding, a $21,000 loss the following year on the care of indigents who comprised 9 per cent of the hospital's patients in 1949, and overall expenses that simply outran income even when, as in 1950, the board sharply increased all of its charges. City council balked, however, at continuing to provide annual subventions to cover these deficits (it now paid, in addition, the full cost of indigent care) while it exercised no effective control (beyond aldermanic and mayoral representation on the board) over hospital expenditures.[20] Meanwhile, Grey County Council, having agreed to assume responsibility for 25 per cent of the G&M's annual deficit in return for four seats on the board and the removal of the surcharge on county patients, refused to accept depreciation as an allowable factor in the calculation of the deficit, an argument that had the effect of reducing the county's liability by 50 per cent.[21] These disputes over the G&M's operating losses were still under negotiation when they were compounded by the announcement, in October 1950, of the Department of Health's much-delayed approval for the expansion of the hospital.[22]

In the end, following 18 months of negotiations with the minister of health, Russell Kelley, and his officials and, no doubt, through the intervention of Kelley's successor, the blunt-speaking 'Mac' Phillips, the department and the board arrived at a compromise. The department agreed to permit the board to add 101 new active-treatment beds (48 private/semi-private, 33 public, and 20 pediatric) and 30 chronic-care beds in return for the abandonment of 76 obsolete beds in the two older wings of the hospital. The end result, a 185-bed hospital, was 20 per cent larger than the department had wanted and 8 per cent smaller than the board's original proposal.[23] In any case, the estimated cost of the project, including new construction, renovations, and equipment, was $2.1 million, triple the cost estimated when the project had first been discussed in 1947. Federal-provincial funding would provide about 20 per cent of the capital required. The remaining 80 per cent, as the board saw it, would be provided in more or less equal shares by Owen Sound on the one hand (42 per cent), and Grey and Bruce counties on the other (38 per cent). Could the municipalities afford it? 'What can a drowning man afford for a life jacket?' the editor of the *Sun-Times* asked on the eve of a referendum to put the question to local ratepayers.[24]

The proposition to raise a million dollars for the G&M through the sale of municipal debentures was defeated on 1 January 1951 by 146 votes.[25] Moreover, the decision of Owen Sound's ratepayers sent a clear message to Grey County Council, who decided at its spring session that the project was too ambitious and that no county funding would be dedicated to it until Owen Sound's contribution was in hand.[26] The hospital's board had hoped that construction would begin in 1951. Now, six months had gone by and the project had not advanced. The board considered two possible courses of action, redrafting a less ambitious project or altering the proposal for city financing. After the annual public meeting of city ratepayers in July 1951 ended in a bitter wrangle over the extent to which higher case loads at the G&M and, consequently, higher expenditures were simply a function of a craze for unnecessary tonsillectomies, the board decided against another referendum in January 1952. With the full support of city council, however, the board of governors launched a major campaign in the spring of 1952 to convince city taxpayers to overturn their narrowly supported earlier decision and approve the sale of municipal debentures to aid the hospital. The campaign pulled out all of the stops, in particular enlisting the city's newspaper and radio station in a massive outpouring of information about the work of the hospital. The newspaper praised the citizens of Owen Sound for being sensibly 'tax conscious' but begged them to exercise their democratic obligation to maintain their hospital as an essential community service. Mayor Sargent took to the airwaves to urge his constituents not to be 'ashamed' at being 'salesmen' for the G&M. City council endorsed the project as an example of Owen Sound's leadership and initiative in matters of civic responsibility. The board promised to adjust the expansion program to whatever funding was eventually available.[27] Nevertheless, the electorate again defeated the proposal, the fourth hospital money by-law to be put before them in six years.[28]

Conditions at the G&M were visibly worsening. By the spring of 1953 all elective surgery had to be cancelled and the waiting list for surgery exceeded 40 cases a month. One hundred and thirteen beds were crammed into space adequate for 80 or 90 at the most. In the oldest wing a bed leg punctured a rotting floor, a symptom of the deterioration that increasingly ate up, in repairs, the now more generous grants distributed annually by the Department of Health for hospital modernization. Clearly some action had to be taken outside the normal mechanisms for obtaining public approval and funding for hospital renovation and expansion. The process started in April 1953 with a request from the minister, Dr Mackinnon Phillips, for a less costly expansion plan. A new proposal emphasizing renovation rather than new construction to achieve a complement of 160–180 beds at a cost of $1.28 million was ready by June and deemed eligible for provincial support of up to 42 per cent of the costs of construction.[29] City council then moved unilaterally, but with the tacit support of the Ontario Municipal Board, to approve a by-law to provide the hospital board, 'in the name of humanitarianism and Christianity,' with $100,000 from the sinking-fund, a $400,000 grant of funds raised from the sale of debentures, and a $150,000 loan. The OMB subsequently held public hearings in Owen Sound to determine the extent of popular opposition to the by-law. Only two citizens spoke against it: representatives of every major industry spoke in support of the scheme. The by-law was approved.[30] City council then added an important condition. Owen Sound's financing was dependent on the availability of funding from Grey and Bruce counties in proportion to their citizens' recent annual utilization of the hospital.

Neither Grey nor Bruce County councils was responsive to the levels of funding proposed by the G&M's board, $210,000 and $70,000 respectively. Grey County Council was favourably disposed towards a grant of just $100,000 because the G&M was only one of six local hospitals (Durham, Mount Forest, Hanover, Markdale, and Meaford were the others) seeking its support. Bruce County was inclined to make a higher contribution to help offset the G&M's annual operating losses, but agreed to consider a capital grant. The board responded by lifting the temporary 15 per cent surcharge on Bruce County patients and reimposing its 15 per cent surcharge on Grey County patients to stimulate their respective councils to make a more generous response.[31] The tactic backfired. Weekly newspapers in both counties raised a hue and cry against the imperiousness of Owen Sounders in general and the G&M in particular. If the G&M was ungrateful for Grey County's offer of $100,000, local editors suggested, so much the better for the area's other hospitals, which were unlikely to find themselves 'sinking in a financial morass' as was the G&M.[32] Bruce County editors complained that the hospital expansion scheme was too 'grand' for Owen Sound's poorer country neighbours, who did not share the city's perception that it was 'the centre of everything.'[33] Bruce County's councillors responded during their spring meeting by refusing to make any grant to the G&M, while their colleagues in Grey tabled the board's request until the surcharge was lifted.[34]

There the matter stood as 1954 drew to a close, four years after the G&M's expansion plans had first been approved, eight years after they had first been discussed. In a last-ditch attempt to salvage the project, the minister himself requested an audience with Grey County councillors in November and begged them to make some gesture that would help him to create a regional 'surgical centre' in Owen Sound for the benefit of the city and both counties without jeopardizing the important role of local hospitals. He suggested a minimum grant of $160,000.[35] This intervention appears to have cleared the way for some fence-mending on the part of Owen

Sound City Council and the G&M's board whose representatives, Mayor Eddie Sargent and Norval Hipwell, reopened negotiations with Grey County Council early in the new year. With the arrival of spring, council agreed to a $160,000 county contribution to the expansion project, payable in four annual instalments of $30,000, with the remaining $40,000 to be raised through a head tax of $1.00 per patient day to be collected from the resident's local municipality. This ensured that the county's northern townships adjacent to Owen Sound paid a proportionately higher share of the total grant. In return the board agreed not only to drop its surcharge on county patients but to refund all surcharges collected since 1952.[36] Bruce County quickly followed suit, guaranteeing a grant of $25,000 and offering to try to raise an additional $25,000 if the board abandoned its surcharge on Bruce patients as well.[37]

With the financing of its expansion program settled, the board moved swiftly to implement its plans, which now called for an additional 72 beds (including new psychiatric and pediatric wards), raising the hospital's total capacity to 169 beds and 33 bassinets. A new operating suite, administrative quarters, an improved kitchen, and general renovations to the 1919 wing were included in the planned expenditure of $1.7 million, which received ministry approval in early October 1955. Construction was barely underway in the spring of 1956 when the ministry provided additional funding to create an outpatients' (emergency) department as well.[38] The official opening of the new northeastern wing in November 1957 in the midst of a howling blizzard brought to a close one of the most difficult chapters in the G&M's long history of attempting to cope with the spiralling demand for hospital care that had been virtually relentless for half a century.

The hospital's latest response was made possible by the historical, if at times unpredictable, interplay of many forces in the community served by the hospital. Ratepayers, local politicians, citizen volunteers, and vested interest groups all played a role in determining the direction and the progress of the debate over the mission of the hospital in post-war society, and the price ultimately to be attached to the presence in their midst of an at least adequate, as defined by modern standards, medical facility. But two new players had entered and influenced the debate. One was the news media. No issue touching on the welfare of local citizens was more widely or thoroughly canvassed on radio or in the local press than the expansion of the hospital. That this coverage almost always supported the G&M's position was partly a tribute to the board's public relations activities, partly the consequence of the involvement of individual representatives of the media in the work of the board, and partly a function of the growing provincial and national debate over the costs of health care that made health questions front-page news in the 1950s. Much of that debate focused on the issue of provincial responsibility for resolving the mounting health care crisis, documented by the Ontario Health Survey Committee in 1950. Thus, quite apart from 'Mac' Phillips's personal and professional interest in a constituency health care issue, the involvement of his ministry, its policy and planning officials, and the provincial treasury in the expansion of the G&M was a sign of the changing attitude at Queen's Park towards social policy questions in general, and health care matters in particular.

It is by no means clear why Leslie Frost who, as treasurer of Ontario, had opposed national hospital insurance became, as premier of Ontario, not only a convert to the idea but its most committed and persuasive champion.[39] Whatever the reason, Frost went to the federal-provincial conference of 1955 determined to pressure the federal government and his fellow premiers, most of whom had lost interest in the national health insurance program first proposed to them by Mackenzie King in 1945, to implement it as soon as possible. It seems to have been the right idea in the right place at the right time. Across Canada patient loads borne by general hospitals had increased about 40 per cent since 1950, but hospital costs per patient day had escalated by 75 per cent in the same period, and the total operating expenses of general hospitals by 260 per cent. One result was that by 1959 public general hospitals like the G&M accounted for three-quarters of all hospital operating expenditures in Canada compared with just 56 per cent in 1922, and only two-thirds of all hospital expenditures as recently as 1952.[40] Frost won the day, and in less than 12 months had approval from his own legislature for an Act to Establish the Hospital Services Commission of Ontario in anticipation of the promulgation, a year later, of the federal government's Hospital Insurance and Diagnostic Services Act.[41] Ottawa's legislation took effect 1 July 1958. Frost's Ontario Hospital Insurance Plan, which the Hospital Services Commission had been set up to administer, came into effect on 1 January 1959.

Ontario's Ministry of Health had been discussing with local hospital boards since 1957 the impact of the introduction of the OHIP in 1959. What was clear to the G&M's governors was that the 1957 expansion of the hospital had merely allowed the board to catch up with existing demand. Any increased use associated with the implementation of universal accessibility would simply lead to a repetition of the hospital's recent accommodation problems, all the more because a thorough inspection of the 1912 wing and the original 1893 building had led to their abandonment once the new addition was completed.[42] Moreover, the RCAF hut (renovated at a cost of $48,000) that now served as a nurses' residence was still inadequate and unusable as a training school facility.

Consequently, the paint was barely dry on the G&M's new wing before the board was laying plans for a subsequent expansion of the hospital's facilities. At the top of the list of priorities, after nearly half a century of half measures to cope with the problem, was a new nurses' residence and training school to accommodate 66 nurses. Replacing the 76 beds abandoned in the two oldest wings was also central to the emerging plan. The major question to be resolved was whether to attempt, once again, to renovate the 1893 and 1912 wings or to demolish them and start again. For reasons of economy the board favoured renovation. The ministry favoured new construction. Architectural surveyors concluded that new construction was less expensive than renovation and recommended demolishing the original hospital building entirely, levelling the 1912 structure to its foundations and rebuilding a new hospital wing on that site, and constructing a new nurses' residence and school just south of the original building. The costs of the project were estimated at $793,000.[43] Compared to the interminable process of securing funding for the most recent expansion of the hospital, financing the next stage promised to be smooth sailing. Government grants totalling $4000 per additional bed were now available subject to the provision that half the new beds had to be restricted to chronic care; there would be, in addition, a provincial contribution to the construction of training school facilities, leaving the board with less than $300,000 to fund.[44]

The architects began to design the two additions in September 1959, but the board, apparently on the strength of nine months of experience with the effects of the Ontario Hospital Insurance Plan, revised its specifications in October. Admissions had increased 13 per cent, average patient stays had crept upward to over 11 days, and usage (an average of 151 patients per day) was once more approaching the hospital's approved capacity (see Table 12). By year's end the local newspaper was again reporting that patients were lodged in hallways and that surgery was being delayed. The impact of OHIP, in short, was immediate, and its effects were not limited to the inflation of utilization statistics. In the first year of the plan's operation, the G&M's income increased 35 per cent. Eighty-four percent of its revenues represented payments made by the province on behalf of insured patients, and a substantial portion of the remainder represented the 50 per cent of income from preferred accommodation charges the hospitals were permitted to retain. For the first time in recent memory the G&M reported a real five-figure surplus.[45] Higher patient demand and better financing argued strongly for a somewhat larger addition than had been originally proposed, and the architects began planning for an 85-bed wing and a 90-bed nurses' residence. This had the effect of pushing the total cost to $1.3 million, the extra financing being split more or less equally between the trust and the Ontario Hospital Services Commission.

What the board could not anticipate was the abrupt increase in construction costs in 1960 (also, apparently, one of the consequences of the advent of administrative centralization[46]) that resulted in all of the tendered bids coming in well above original estimates. To stay within the project's approved budget, the board was forced at the last minute to pare 12 beds from the plan before letting the contract in late November 1960.[47] A year later, the nurses' residence and training school was complete and occupied. Construction on the new wing began in the spring of 1962 when two local labourers,

TABLE 12
Summary data, G&M Hospital, 1949-64

|  | 1949 | 1950 | 1951 | 1952 | 1953 | 1954 | 1955 |
|---|---|---|---|---|---|---|---|
| No. of bed patients | 3,457 | 3,882 | 4,015 | 4,032 | 4,151 | 4,198 | 4,131 |
| Average stay (days) | 8.9 | 9.1 | 9.1 | 9.0 | 8.9 | 8.9 | 9.0 |
| Avg. no. of patients/day | 101 | 97 | 100 | 100 | 101 | 103 | 103 |
| No. of births | 667 | 630 | 646 | 667 | 671 | 658 | 635 |
| No. of operations | 2,452 | 2,088 | 2,317 | 2,252 | 2,252 | 2,300 | 2,492 |
| No. of x-ray patients | 4,928 | 5,247 | 5,728 | 5,664 | 10,039 | 8,450 | 8,617 |
| No. of lab procedures | 9,643 |  | 13,348 |  | 15,710 | 16,137 |  |
| No. of outpatients |  |  |  |  | 6,205 |  | 6,000 |
| Profit/(loss) ($) | (43,241.00) | (7,500.00) | (11,356.00) | (6,828.00) | (7,000.00) | (4,961.00) | 14,530.00 |

|  | 1956 | 1957 | 1958 | 1959 | 1963 | 1964 |
|---|---|---|---|---|---|---|
| No. of bed patients |  | 4,308 | 4,511 | 4,959 | 5,807 | 5,494 |
| Average stay (days) |  | 8.9 | 10.4 | 10.2 | 11.3 |  |
| Avg. no. of patients/day |  | 106 | 125 | 151 | 182 | 206 |
| No. of births | 679 | 679 | 653 | 620 | 182 | 206 |
| No. of operations | 2,591 | 2,361 | 2,110 |  | 2,696 | 2,821 |
| No. of x-ray patients | 6,967 | 8,091 | 5,547 |  | 2,696 | 2,821 |
| No. of lab procedures | 39,979 | 27,243 | 29,556 |  |  |  |
| No. of outpatients |  |  | 2,459 |  | 4,118 | 4,263 |
| Profit/(loss) ($) |  | (29,814.66) | (21,008.00) | 16,460.00 | 39,511.00 | 45,855.00 |

SOURCES: G&M Annual Reports; Owen Sound *Daily Sun-Times*

Frank Jones and David Gagan, dug by hand a 360-cubic-foot bore hole for the contractor. When no evidence of quicksand or underground streams was found, the project proceeded to a successful conclusion in March 1963, the addition having been restored to its originally planned 85 beds.[48]

The General and Marine Hospital was now, to all intents and purposes, a wholly new facility. Its 244 beds (75 medical, 84 surgical, 26 obstetric, 34 chronic, 25 pediatric) were a long-overdue solution to a historical problem that had taken nearly two decades to resolve, while its new outpatient, cardiology, and physiotherapy departments and its monthly cancer clinic were important manifestations of the very latest developments in diagnostic, preventative, and rehabilitation medicine. It was also a completely new enterprise in another sense. In 1956, 97 per cent of the G&M's revenue had been derived from the fees of paying patients. In 1963, 97 per cent of its revenue came from the Province of Ontario in the form of reimbursements for the treatment of insured patients at rates geared to the cost of operating the hospital. The board began to enjoy, briefly, the benefits of budgetary processes that allowed for advanced planning and resulted in annual surpluses which could be used to improve the hospital's equipment and operations.

These surpluses were also evidence, however, of the massive growth in the volume of health care delivered and the parallel growth of expenditures on hospital facilities and care engendered first by the appearance of voluntary prepaid health insurance schemes and then by the provinces' hospital insurance plans. Across Canada the volume of hospital care delivered by public general hospitals increased 56 per cent between 1948 and 1958, and 27 per cent between 1958 and 1962. Before 1958 the increase in volume of care was attributable almost entirely to rates of utilization: after 1958 it was compounded by lengthening stays.[49] One reason for this shift was that individual patients no longer faced a dire personal financial penalty for hospitalization prolonged in the interest of complete recovery. A second reason was the growing trend, with the advent of provincial hospital insurance in particular, for physicians to hospitalize patients for observation and diagnosis. Paralleling this increase in the volume of bed care delivered was a similar explosion of outpatient services, which rapidly replaced physicians' surgeries and house calls as the source not only of emergency treatment but increasingly of very routine medical inquiries.[50]

All of these factors can be seen in the impact of OHIP on the G&M. In the first week of the plan's operation the hospital provided care to a number of patients (157), 90 per cent of whom were insured under the new program.[51] In the first year of the insurance plan's operation, the number of inpatients treated increased 13 per cent, but their average stay was extended only marginally, from 10.2 to 10.4 days. (See Table 12.) By 1963 the combination of a 33 per cent increase in cases since 1958 and stays that now averaged more than 11 days meant that in a single year the G&M logged as many treatment days as it had in the period 1893–1906. The number of patients admitted in 1963 was equal to the number admitted between 1 October 1893 and 30 September 1915. The reasons for their admission to the hospital also reflected broader provincial and national patterns. As Table 13 indicates, medical and pediatric (children under 15 years of age) patients represented a significantly higher proportion of cases in 1963 than they had a decade earlier. In part this was a function of the redistribution of the hospital's beds during expansion and renovation; but it also reflects the growing number of admissions for diagnostic purposes and the emerging focus of medical treatment on two demographic sectors of society, the very young and the sick, often chronically ill, elderly.[52]

With the advent of universally accessible hospital care, the Owen Sound General and Marine Hospital had become a 'centre for major surgery, and for advanced diagnostic and treatment facilities' as its promoters had intended when they launched their rebuilding program a decade earlier. Under the impact of universal accessibility as defined by the province's new hospital insurance plan, however, it was a centre that in 1963 was already inadequate and would be rendered almost completely obsolete with the introduction of universal medical insurance in July 1968. The stage was set for the implementation of the second phase of the federal government's health care program when the Medical Care Act was passed in 1966 and brought into effect two years later, largely over the objections of

TABLE 13
Cases treated, G&M Hospital, 1950-63 (percentages)

|  | 1950 | 1951 | 1960 |
|---|---|---|---|
| Medical | 16.7 | 15.7 | 22.3 |
| Surgical | 23.3 | 23.7 | 14.3 |
| Gynecology | 5.1 | 5.3 | 5.3 |
| Orthopedic | 3.6 | 3.8 | 3.7 |
| Obstetric | 17.9 | 17.9 | 15.4 |
| Newborn | 16.2 | 16.0 | 13.4 |
| Pediatric | 6.3 | 6.3 | 19.5 |
| Eye/ear/nose | 10.9 | 11.2 | 6.0 |

SOURCE: Monthly Analyses of Hospital Service, G&M Hospital, Miscellaneous Reports

the medical profession and in spite of misgivings on the part of provincial governments, all of which, nevertheless had implemented medical care insurance schemes by 1971.[54]

If the subsequent experience of the Owen Sound General and Marine Hospital is an accurate indicator of the effects of universal access to both hospitalization and physicians' services, those misgivings were well-placed in both the short and the long term. Even before the advent of universal medical care, in fact as soon as the 1963 addition had been completed, the seemingly insatiable demand for the hospital's services compelled the board to reassess its priorities. The review took the form of a year-long survey of the hospital's needs in relation to current and projected usage. The survey concluded that within a year of reconstruction the G&M had again reached capacity in its medical, surgical, and pediatrics departments. Demand for accommodation for the chronically ill in particular could no longer be met. Only obstetrics had experienced a decline in admissions. To meet current demand, a minimum of 36 additional beds was required immediately, and in the long term nearly 100. As well, the G&M's laundry, cafeteria, laboratory, and pharmacy facilities and its electrical substation would have to be expanded, while the medical staff was lobbying for larger outpatient facilities and for an intensive care unit as part of any proposed construction program. The costs of the project were estimated at $1.8 million without additional beds, $4.1 million with 58 additional beds.[55] After 18 months of deliberation and informal consultation with the Ontario Hospital Services Commission, the board of governors approved in principle a two-stage construction program for presentation to the ministry.[56]

There were, however, three major obstacles to be overcome. First, there was no space left on the old Brownlee site for expansion (additional automobile parking areas were already being created at the expense of a long-established residential neighbourhood). More critically, expansion would require additional medical and professional nursing staff, but even before expansion was approved it had been widely acknowledged that Owen Sound had a severe shortage of physicians and graduate nurses. In an effort to attract qualified nurses, the board implemented wage parity with Metropolitan Toronto hospitals and a staff evaluation/merit system for non-unionized employees in order to recruit and retain other skilled health care workers. But remuneration was not the only stumbling block to the recruitment of the necessary staff. Recent graduates of nursing schools were in short supply. To enhance both the number and the qualifications of nursing graduates the province turned to its new community college system as the provider of nursing education. For example, the G&M's training school was transferred in 1967 to Georgian College. Meanwhile, the available pool consisted primarily of inactive women with families for whom there was neither adequate housing nor daycare facilities in Owen Sound. The board seriously considered, as many other hospitals were doing, providing both subsidized housing and child care in an effort to induce these women to re-enter the workforce.[57] The plan proved unworkable, and in 1967 the board was forced to close 20 chronic care beds because of staff shortages. Nevertheless, in a single year the hospital's wage bill, representing 70 per cent of the G&M's total 1967 operating budget, increased $400,000. This scenario, repeated throughout the Ontario health care system, created the third hurdle to expansion, the growing alarm at Queen's Park over the escalating costs of providing universal accessibility not only to hospital but, commencing in 1968, to medical services as well.

After two years of delays, the Ontario Hospital Services Commission refused, in March 1969, to approve the G&M's expansion plans as part of a larger policy decision to restrict the growth of the province's health care budget, which was expected, even with the implementation of funding controls, to reach $1.5 billion by the middle of the next decade.[58] An expanded outpatient department and a modest coronary care unit represented the ministry's only concessions to the G&M's now completely overtaxed and largely unworkable facilities.[59] The only light on the horizon was the promise of yet another planning exercise to promote, in entirely new circumstances, the age-old goal of the hospital as a public charity – efficiency – to justify the continued support of its mentors.

Like its sister public general hospitals in Ontario, the General and Marine Hospital had emerged in 1945 from the era of depression and war to face an unprecedented demand for its services. The demand came, in unequal proportions, from its historical clientele. Indigent patients dependent on municipal charity for medical care and treated by the hospital below cost continued to account for about 10 per cent of all patients and a disproportionate share of total days of care given. Paying 'patients of moderate means,' who since the 1920s had borne the brunt of hospital operating costs in the form of higher maintenance fees and service charges, and who had rejected hospital care as far as possible during the Depression, reappeared in even larger numbers after the war as beneficiaries of voluntary group hospitalization insurance. Demand and the higher costs it entailed for expansion, labour, and the latest developments in diagnostic and therapeutic care quickly outran the hospital's ability to cope with the financial consequences of this second revolution in hospital-based medicine. At the same time, public sympathy for and philanthropy towards the hospital, now increasingly identified as a business rather than a charity, had never been at a lower ebb.

Caught between the millstones of public demand for its services and lack of public interest in its problems, the G&M endured a long and exhausting local political struggle for survival between 1947 and 1957, mirroring the national and provincial debates over the implementation of social policies delayed since the onset of the war. The advent of national health insurance abruptly redefined the G&M's mission and prospects for survival. It did not reduce the magnitude of the G&M's problems. For 40 years the public general hospitals of Ontario had grappled autonomously and independently, as charitable institutions, with the problem of gearing their services to the needs of paying patients in order to generate the income necessary to provide adequate medical care for all members of the community. As the impact of universal accessibility was swiftly unleashed, the local hospital's new role as a self-governing charity in a highly centralized health care system soon became evident. Its task was now to mediate, through the imaginative deployment of both its public and private assets, the problem of too many people competing for too few health care resources as defined by the limits of society's ability to pay, through taxation, for universal accessibility. Voluntary medical philanthropy had come full circle. The G&M had begun its existence as a place where the affluent provided medical charity for the poor. Later, in the 1920s, patients who could afford medical care subsidized the treatment of those who could not. Now, the healthy subsidized the sick[60] in a new era of rising popular expectations about the availability and the therapeutic potential of hospital-centred medical care, and rising political anxiety about the costs of fulfilling those expectations.

# 6
# 'Once Upon a Time There Was No Frank Miller'

The provincial government's fear that the introduction in October 1969 of Ontario's medical care plan would create, rather than remove, an economic barrier to health care availability soon became a reality. Between 1972 and 1976 gross expenditures on health care in Ontario increased 104 per cent. The greatest single component of these costs was rising expenditures on hospitals, which accounted, by the mid-1970s, for 53 per cent of the province's health care budget.[1] The legislature's Select Committee on Health Care Financing and Costs traced the source of these rapidly escalating hospital costs to high utilization rates relative to the number of beds available. Of Canada's 10 provinces, Ontario had the second lowest ratio of hospital beds per capita and one of the highest occupancy rates, producing an intensity of usage that sustained – largely through wage costs – one of the most expensive hospital systems in the country.[2] Other observers viewing these developments found different explanations. For example, Canadians, by the mid-1970s, had the highest rate of hospitalization in the western world, much of it associated with life-style-induced degenerative diseases which contributed to a 'literally unlimited' demand for marginally useful but extremely costly care.[3] More generally, students of medical ethics had become concerned that modern society's 'sense of the fragility of human existence ... [had been] reduced to a hope in immortality' through medical technology, whatever the cost.[4] Wherever the problem lay, its solution rested squarely with the provincial government.

The government's short-term solution was to cut costs while preserving accessibility. As early as 1969, major hospital construction projects were put on hold indefinitely. The next phase involved holding the line on increases in hospital operating budgets, first by restricting the rate of growth of new services, then by slashing budgets, and finally, under Conservative Premier William Davis's health minister, Frank Miller, closing not only wards but entire hospitals. Under these draconian conditions the G&M, which experienced a 28 per cent increase in annual inpatient admissions between 1968 and 1972, experienced even more difficult sledding as it cut back staff and services to avoid (not always successfully) annual operating deficits on shrinking budgets. By 1972 physicians were being actively discouraged from making 'speculative' admissions in an effort to free beds for the waiting-list of 290 surgical cases and to get bedridden patients out of the hospital's corridors. In 1974 tonsillectomies were removed from the list of approved hospital procedures. By 1975 the hospital could no longer accommodate the demand for chronic care, some of its most essential services – the pharmacy, laboratory, and radiology departments – were unable to function effectively in their existing quarters, surgical bookings had become 'a hopeless mess,' and staff reductions were made to meet ministry-imposed budget targets.[5] The frustrations of the board, the staff, and the patients were summed up by a local historian who began a retrospective article on the origins of the hospital with a comment on the current state of affairs. 'Once upon a time there was no Frank Miller, no closing of hospitals, no shutting down of wards and cutting beds, no reducing budgets. Once upon a time,' he recalled, 'there was a small hospital in the growing city of Owen Sound that had more than enough beds for all of its patients.'[6] In 1976, 1886 or, for that matter, 1936 was ancient, perhaps even mythological, history. The relevant past was the brief, shining moment – in 1963, perhaps – when everyone who wanted to be hospitalized was.

The G&M's board of governors had little choice but to attempt to cope, on an ad hoc basis, with its rapidly accumulating problems. Some relief was provided in 1975 when the OHSC approved the installation of portable buildings to accommodate expanded laboratory, pharmacy, and nuclear medicine facilities, but this temporary expansion and renovation program was insignificant in comparison with the staggering underfunding the hospital endured for the remainder of the decade. Two developments, however, one short term, the other long range, provided some reasons, amidst this crisis, for optimism about the future of the hospital.

The first of these developments was the provincial government's decision to strive for rationalization, efficiency, and economy in the distribution and utilization of health care resources on a regional basis by implementing a process of decentralized planning carried out by district planning councils representing hospital users, health care providers, local government, and the ministry. In fact, as early as 1967 the ministry of health had advised the G&M's board that it proposed to create a Grey-Bruce Health Services Planning Committee in order to achieve 'total utilization of hospital beds and more economical use of existing equipment and ... ancillary services' in the twin counties.[7] The initial meeting of the committee did not take place, however, until June 1971. In the meantime, the OHSC had designated the General and Marine as a 'district' hospital, and following the first meeting of the committee (later the District Health Council), the board was invited by the ministry to submit a long-range master plan defining the role that an expanded G&M would play in a regional health care system.[8] The board immediately contracted with Woods, Gordon Company of Toronto to develop their plan, which was presented to the ministry in the summer of 1972 and which ultimately envisaged the expansion of the G&M to a 355-bed hospital. Although it approved of the plan in principle, the hospital commission's immediate reaction was that the proposed expansion was too conservative, that a 550-bed hospital was more appropriate for the region's future needs. As it happened, the commission's estimate was the more realistic one, if only because the minister subsequently intervened to forestall any expansion until the end of the decade and to insist on a planning horizon that extended well into the 1980s. He and his officials raised the interesting possibility, however, of merging the operations of the G&M and the provincially operated Mackinnon Phillips Psychiatric Hospital on the city's eastern outskirts, where ample land for expansion was available.[9]

This was in 1974. Events moved somewhat more quickly than the ministry had predicted, however, largely because the impetus for the regional rationalization of health care services gathered momentum as the funding crisis, and its political fall-out, worsened. By 1976 the ministry had created 15 district health councils (17 more were planned) with the responsibility to evaluate and recommend ways of meeting the 'total health care' needs of their respective populations within the context of the government's program of fiscal restraint.[10] In the case of Grey and Bruce counties, the problems were particularly thorny. A widely dispersed, largely rural population relied on several very small local cottage hospitals (Durham, Chesley, Mount Forest, Wiarton, Southampton, Lion's Head, Kincardine), two mid-sized (Hanover, Walkerton) subregional hospitals, and one district hospital (the G&M) for different levels of hospital care; but the threatened loss of any of these facilities, or their inability to acquire at least some essential medical specialization, was a potential source of animosity towards the G&M as in the past. Nevertheless, the district health council eventually endorsed a plan whereby a completely new regional health centre in Owen Sound would provide specialized hospital and medical services for the two counties, whose population, excluding Owen Sound, already accounted for nearly 40 per cent of the G&M's annual patient load. Local hospitals would become convalescent facilities to permit patients able to leave the regional hospital, but still requiring convalescent care, to recover in community health care centres close to their families.[11]

In the end, the G&M's board proposed, and the DHC endorsed, the construction of a new 450-bed facility estimated to cost $35 million, of which $8 million was to be raised from municipal grants and at least $2 million from public subscriptions. In spite of initial apprehensions whether a fund-raising appeal could succeed, the campaign, led by hospital staff, board members, and volunteers, and supported by local government and industry, raised in excess of $16 million dollars, a convincing demonstration that the hospital was still the single most important secular charity in the community.

The new Grey Bruce Regional Health Centre replaced the General and Marine Hospital in 1985, exactly one century after the need for a hospital was first articulated by the citizens of Owen Sound.

The second development that facilitated the G&M's metamorphosis was the ministry's decision to agree to a merger of the G&M and Mackinnon Phillips hospitals in 1978. For 15 years the G&M's most pressing problem had been the lack of adequate chronic care facilities. As early as 1974, transferring the G&M's chronic patients to the underutilized psychiatric facility had been proposed, and acknowledged by the ministry, as a potential solution. After two years of informal discussions, the ministry and the board exchanged letters of intent in 1976, and in 1977 the province formally agreed to merge the Mackinnon Phillips and G&M operations under a single corporation in 1978. Moreover, in light of the developing plan for a new regional health centre, the ministry subsequently sold the psychiatric facility to the G&M's board for $1.00, effectively providing the G&M, at the same time and at no cost, with the land (66 acres) it needed for expansion whenever ministry approval was forthcoming.[12] Plans were made to transfer chronic patients to the psychiatric facility and, as a stopgap measure, to make temporary repairs and alterations to the G&M to extend its life until the new regional health centre was approved, funded, and constructed.

The sod was turned for the new hospital on 26 July 1983, and the tender was let eight months later. When the Grey Bruce Regional Health Centre was complete, the G&M was sold, to be converted into apartments, and a century-old record of service came to an end. It had begun in 1893 partly in response to the fear of epidemic disease, and partly as a symbol of civic progressivism. Primarily, however, the General and Marine Hospital expressed the community's social and moral obligation to provide care for strangers and for the homeless sick poor in a setting where their convalescence or death would take place in a domestic atmosphere defined by Christian humanitarianism. Within a decade this custodial function had begun to give way to a higher therapeutic objective promoted by the advent of safe aseptic surgery, by the growing demand for hospital-centred obstetric care, by the transformation of nursing from a domestic into a medical science, and above all, perhaps, by the new scientific imperatives of the rising medical profession for whom hospitals had become the institutional symbols of their special calling. Better care and higher survival rates increasingly attracted the attention of middle-class patients who traditionally had been treated at home but who were now willing to be hospitalized and to pay for preferential care in private or semi-private rooms. The expansion of the G&M in 1911–12 reflected both the growing demand for hospitalization by paying patients and the determination of the medical staff to transform the hospital into a centre for the active treatment of disease using their newly acquired diagnostic and surgical skills.

That transformation was more or less complete by 1930. It was characterized in particular by the overwhelming preponderance of surgical and obstetrics cases among the hospital's patients, by the growing proportion of female patients, and by the hospital's almost total dependence for its financial stability on the fees of paying patients willing to be hospitalized at prices they could afford for preferential care. In the 1920s the G&M could boast that it was not unlike a hotel, with a wide range of services geared to the guest's ability to pay, where all members of the community could reap the benefits of modern medical efficiency. Whether all patients saw the hospital in this light is not clear, but it is certain that by 1930 birth, acute sickness, and, to a lesser extent, death were increasingly being transferred from the home to the hospital.

The second modernization of the G&M in 1929 was an accommodation of this trend. The cost of removing these events to the hospital, however, was significant. Most paying patients paid a maintenance premium to avoid the historical social stigma of the public wards. As municipal and provincial subventions increasingly fell behind the spiralling price of maintaining the sick poor amid the costly complexity of the modern medical workshop, the premium increased to include the cost of medical charity. Even under the best economic conditions, the assumption that paying patients could, or would, shoulder for very long the burden of society's obligations to the sick poor was questionable, given the rate at which the cost of scientific medicine was advancing. The Great Depression effectively submerged that assumption in a flood of human misery which quickly disabused the middle classes in particular of their belief that a health care system rooted in the ability to pay was preferable to a system in which medical necessity was the first criterion of accessibility. As the Depression deepened, paying patients resisted hospitalization at any cost, and the G&M quickly reverted to its original role as a dispenser of medical charity.

The appearance of voluntary hospital insurance during the Second World War and its widespread availability after the war, post-war population growth, and the acquisition of drugs such as penicillin by civilian hospitals regenerated and accelerated demand for hospital care after 1945. For the G&M, coping with this demand involved the deployment of resources – additional beds, more qualified nurses, a larger lay workforce, a greater array of resident medical specialists, more modern equipment – it could acquire only by increasing its revenues. The only source of that additional income was the paying (or at least insured) patient who was still paying twice for hospital care, once for himself and once for his less affluent neighbour whose public ward bed was subsidized well below the hospital's actual cost of treatment. Under such conditions taxpayers were reluctant to accede to further voluntary taxation to sustain the G&M's seemingly endless need for support: hence the prolonged debate in Owen Sound, between 1947 and 1955, over responsibility for the socially essential, but politically contentious, expansion of hospital facilities. One solution was a hospital care system which guaranteed accessibility, on the same basis, to all and spread the costs equitably among all users. The introduction of such a system in 1958 was largely the result of the historical experience of the Canadian middle classes not only as users, but as the inventors of the modern hospital and, for thirty years, the principal promoters and beneficiaries of its scientific promise.

The advent of national hospital insurance may have solved the ancient problem of providing medical philanthropy for the poor, but in communities like Owen Sound it solved the much more recent and equally urgent problem of preventing the medical impoverishment of paying patients. By the 1950s they were confronted with the insecurity represented by unanticipated hospitalization in medically and socially essential institutions which they were obliged to build, maintain, and subsidize with their incomes, but whose necessary services they could no longer afford. Universal accessibility to hospital care after 1 January 1959, and to medical care a decade later, presented both a solution and new challenges. The extra case load generated by newly insured patients, the trend towards longer hospital stays, the growing frequency of admission for observation and diagnosis, and the sky-rocketing costs of medical technology severely taxed the hospital's increasingly restricted resources until, in recognition of its essential mission among a large regional population, the government of Ontario at last permitted the G&M to fulfil its promise in a new guise.

Through all of these developments the General and Marine Hospital was nurtured, supported, and promoted by many people. Between 1891 and 1963 the citizens of Owen Sound and Grey and Bruce counties, individually and through their elected councils and voluntary organizations, contributed more than $1 million to hospital construction projects alone. From 1903 until 1950 the hospital's domestic requirements were largely met by the efforts of the hospital auxiliary. For example, between 1918 and 1928, when there were no extraordinary fund-raising activities, the auxiliary contributed more than $20,000 to the hospital. After 1950 this fund-raising ability – now directed towards the acquisition of new equipment – was combined with direct hospital voluntarism (1500 hours a month by the 1970s) to improve the quality of patients' stays. Physicians and nurses, quite apart from their responsibility for the well-being of individual patients, were also concerned with the G&M's institutional development as a health care centre. Standardization, technological innovations such as the introduction of x-ray diagnosis and therapy, improved neo-natal facilities in the 1930s, a major campaign in the 1940s to educate expectant mothers and reduce the incidence of infant mortality, the relentless push for a broader representation of medical specialization in the G&M since the 1950s, and the implementation of the medical 'team' concept in the 1970s are all examples of initiatives promoted by the medical staff to ensure that the G&M kept pace with the progress of medical science.

Marshalling all of this activity into a coherent program of patient care consistent with the hospital's resource base was a long succession of very able superintendents and nursing supervisors whose credentials as professional hospital administrators represented, more often than not, a process of baptism under fire in the trench warfare of medical philanthropy. The foundation on which the enterprise was ultimately erected, however, was the historical steadfastness of the citizen volunteers who, as members of the hospital trust and its board, promoted the interests of the hospital, in the words of one of its founders, as 'an indispensable necessity among us.' This is not to undervalue the contribution of the nurses, physicians, superintendents, or lay personnel whose own developing professionalism was largely the source of the hospital's transformation from an almshouse into a rigorously disciplined instrument of scientific medical care. Nevertheless, whatever their individual motives may have been, collectively, three or four generations of like-minded citizens managed to respond successfully to the health care needs and priorities of the population of two counties by sustaining, through good times and bad, with or without popular support, for a hundred years, the work of the Owen Sound General and Marine Hospital. It was a formidable task even in the best of times. Their objective was to 'Heal The Sick.' Striving for it always demanded, in St Paul's words, that they 'be not weary in well-doing.'

APPENDIX I

# Lady Superintendents and Administrators, Owen Sound General and Marine Hospital, 1893–1985

**Lady Superintendents:**

| | |
|---|---|
| J.E. Moore | 1893 |
| E. McKenzie | 1894–9 |
| E. Hunter | 1899–1904 |
| Jessie Duncan | 1904–9 |
| Margaret Carson | 1909–11 |
| M. Redmond | 1911–14 |
| Ethel Wood | 1914–18 |
| Jennie McArthur | 1918–24 |
| Georgina Thompson | 1924–5 |
| Maud Sterling | 1925–8 |
| Edith Jefferies | 1928–9 |
| Mabel Sharp | 1919–30 |
| Bertha Hall | 1930–7 |
| Pearl Morrison | 1937 |
| Rahno Beamish | 1937–40 |
| Reta Brown | 1941–7 |

**Administrators:**

| | |
|---|---|
| James Clark | 1941–76 |
| A.L. McIntosh | 1976–81 |
| G.A. Pierce | 1981– |

APPENDIX II

# Board Presidents, Owen Sound General and Marine Hospital Trust

| | |
|---|---|
| S.J. Parker | 1893–7, 1899 |
| Allan Cameron | 1898, 1902–5 |
| J. McLauchlan | 1899–1902, 1906 |
| John Armstrong | 1907–9 |
| J.M. Kilbourn | 1910–12 |
| F.W. Harrison | 1913–15 |
| Judge Widdifield | 1915–17 |
| Rev. Thurlow Fraser | 1918 |
| Elias Lemon | 1919–20 |
| Joseph McLinden | 1921–37 |
| Dr G.W. Holmes | 1937–44 |
| Neil Kennedy | 1945–8 |
| James Garvie | 1949–50 |
| Dr George McKee | 1951–2 |
| Norval Hipwell | 1953 |
| Arthur Marron | 1954–7 |
| Mrs W.P. Telford | 1958, 1965–66 |
| William Hawken | 1959–62 |
| Howard Hindman | 1963–4, 1976–7 |
| M.A. Craig | 1967–8, 1972–5 |
| Harold Van Wyck | 1969–71 |
| J.A. Kirby | 1978–81 |
| B.R. Price | 1982–3 |
| R.A. Morrison | 1984–5 |

# Notes

CHAPTER 1

1 Owen Sound *Times*, 22 June 1893
2 This summary reflects the arguments fully developed in Jacob Spelt, *Urban Developement in South-Central Ontario* (Toronto 1972), especially chs. 4 and 5; John McCallum, *Unequal Beginnings: Agriculture and Economic Development in Quebec and Ontario until 1870* (Toronto 1980), especially ch. 7; David Gagan, *Hopeful Travellers: Families, Land, and Social Change in Mid-Victorian Peel County, Canada West* (Toronto 1981), esp. chs. 5 and 6; and Morris Zaslow, *The Opening of the Canadian North, 1870–1914* (Toronto 1971), ch. 7.
3 Owen Sound *Times*, 18 July 1889 (a 'Short History' of Owen Sound for a convention of Freemasons)
4 William Taylor (Woodlands, Manitoba) to editor, Brampton *Times*, 29 Aug. 1874, describes in detail this journey taken by his family and many of his neighbours.
5 Unless otherwise noted, the economic and demographic data cited in this and the following discussion are drawn from the published *Census of Canada, 1891* (Ottawa 1893); Province of Ontario, Legislative Assembly, *Sessional Papers*, Report of the Registrar-General (henceforward cited as OSP); and assessment, shipping, and other reports gleaned from the surviving Owen Sound newspapers. T.A. Davidson, *A New History of Grey County* (Owen Sound 1972), especially chs. 31, 35–7, and 41, contains much interesting anecdotal material.
6 Pierre Berton, *The Last Spike: The Great Railway, 1881–1885* (Toronto 1971), 270–1
7 Owen Sound *Times*, 30 July 1891
8 Ibid., 18 July 1889
9 Ibid., 6 Dec. 1888, 24 Jan. 1889

10 These ideas are discussed in Ramsay Cook, *The Regenerators: Social Criticism in Late Victorian English Canada* (Toronto 1985).
11 See, for example, Desmond Morton, *Mayor Howland, The Citizens' Candidate* (Toronto 1973).
12 Owen Sound *Times*, 1 Nov. 1888
13 This information is drawn largely from an extensive set of newspaper clippings on the history of Owen Sound collected by Miss Izetta Fraser.
14 Joseph Schull, *Ontario since 1867* (Toronto 1978), 88
15 Andrew Jones and Leonard Rutman, *In the Children's Aid: J.J. Kelso and Child Welfare in Ontario* (Toronto 1981), 81
16 United Church Archives, Biographical Files, Sara Brackbill and Retta Gifford Kilbourn
17 Louis A. Wood, in *A History of Farmers' Movements in Canada*, ed. F.J. Griezic (Toronto 1975), 71–83
18 See R.B. Splane, *Social Welfare in Ontario, 1791–1893* (Toronto 1965), 198; J.T. Phair, 'Public Health in Ontario,' *The Development of Public Health in Canada*, ed. R.D. Defries (Toronto 1940), 67.
19 See Gretchen Condran and Eileen Crimmins-Gardner, 'Public Health Measures and Mortality in U.S. Cities in the Late Nineteenth Century,' *Human Ecology*, 6 (1978):27–54
20 Owen Sound *Times*, 7 Feb. 1887, 1 Nov. 1888, 31 May 1894, 27 Feb. 1896
21 Ibid., 20 Feb. 1908
22 Owen Sound General and Marine Hospital, *Annual Report*, 1904 (henceforward cited as *Annual Report*)
23 Owen Sound *Times*, 19 Sept. 1891
24 Ibid., 21 Jan. 1889, 25 May 1893
25 For the history of voluntary hospitals in the early nineteenth century see George Rosen, 'The Hospital: Historical Sociology of a Community Institution,' in *The Hospital in Modern Society*, ed. Eliot Friedson (London 1963), 24–5; Noel Parry and José Parry, *The Rise of the Medical Profession: A Study of Collective Mobility* (London 1976), 136–7, 181; Morris J. Vogel, *The Invention of the Modern Hospital: Boston, 1870–1930* (Chicago 1980), 1–28; Charles E. Rosenberg, 'Inward Vision and Outward Glance: The Shaping of the American Hospital, 1880–1914,' in *Social History and Social Policy*, ed. David J. Rothman and Stanton Wheeler (New York 1981), 19; Brian Abel-Smith, *The Hospitals, 1800–1948: A Study in Social Administration in England and Wales* (London 1964), esp. chs. 1–7.
26 Paul Starr, *The Social Transformation of American Medicine* (New York 1982), 146
27 Ibid., 146–59; Abel-Smith, chs. 5, 9; Vogel, 60–7; John V. Pickstone, *Medicine and Industrial Society: A History of Hospital Development in Manchester and Its Region, 1752–1946* (Manchester 1985), esp. ch. 9
28 Vogel, 77
29 Paul Starr, 'Medicine, Economy and Society in Nineteenth-Century America,'

in *The Medicine Show*, ed. Patricia Branca (New York 1977), 47
30 Rosenberg, 'Inward Vision, Outward Glance,' 24–33; Starr, *Social Transformation*, 161–78; Rosen, 'The Hospital,' 26–30
31 Vogel, 135; Starr, 'Medicine, Economy and Society in Nineteenth Century America,' 58–60
32 OSP, 1891, no. 10, Inspector of Prisons and Charities
33 Ibid.
34 W.G. Crosbie, *The Toronto General Hospital, 1819–1965: A Chronicle* (Toronto 1975) 68–106
35 'Hospitals, Government Establishments,' *Canadian Lancet*, 10 (Aug. 1878):376–7
36 'The Pay System at Hospitals,' *Canadian Lancet*, 27 (Dec. 1894):126–7; 'Medical Libraries, Their Development and Use,' ibid., 28 (April 1896):83–4; 'Hospitals and the Medical Profession,' ibid., 41 (Sept. 1907):71–1; 'Some Hospital Problems,' ibid., 41 (Feb. 1908):465–6; "Hospitals and City Life,' ibid., 42 (Feb. 1909):403–4
37 Owen Sound *Times*, 15, 31 Jan. 1889
38 Ibid., 14 Feb. 1889
39 Ibid., 28 Feb. 1895; Owen Sound *Advertiser*, 20 Oct. 1899; Davidson, 323
40 Owen Sound General and Marine Hospital, Board of Trustees, Minute Books, 3 June 1891 (henceforward cited as Minutes)
41 Minutes, 28 Sept. 1891
42 Minutes, 3, 11 June, 5, 6, 12, 17 Aug., 8 Sept. 1891; Owen Sound *Times*, 4 June, 24 Sept. 1891. An interesting footnote to all of this activity is that, for reasons that remain clouded in obscurity, the hospital trust's application for incorporation was never officially recorded as having been approved by the lieutenant-governor-in-council, and in 1965 a private member's bill had to be enacted by the Legislature of Ontario to incorporate the Owen Sound General and Marine Hospital.
43 Minutes, 16 Oct., 5 Nov., 9 Dec. 1891, 5, 12, 13 Jan., 11, 12 March 1892
44 OSP, 1894, no. 24, Inspector of Prisons and Charities; Ontario Department of Health, *The Hospitals of Ontario: A Short History* (Toronto 1934), 17–18
45 Minutes, 6, 8, 21 May, 1, 19, 30 June, 13 July 1893; Owen Sound *Times*, 25 May, 1 June 1893
46 *By-Laws and Rules and Regulations of the Owen Sound General and Marine Hospital* (Owen Sound, 11 April 1891), 1–7, 9–11
47 Rosen, 'The Hospital,' 28; Rosenberg, 'Inward Vision,' 33; Abel-Smith, 68; John Woodward, *To Do the Sick No Harm: A Study of the British Voluntary Hospital System to 1875* (London 1974), 29–35
48 Minutes, 22 Aug., 3 Oct. 1893
49 Ibid., 23 Nov. 1893
50 Ibid., 2 Dec. 1893
51 OSP, 1890, no. 10, Inspector of Prisons and Charities

52 OSP, 1885, no. 39, Inspector of Prisons and Charities
53 OSP, 1890, no. 14, Inspector of Prisons and Charities
54 Ibid.
55 Owen Sound *Times*, 11 Jan. 1894
56 Minutes, 9 May 1894
57 The foregoing discussion is based on an analysis of the G&M's *Rules and Regulations*.
58 *By-Laws of the Owen Sound General and Marine Hospital Trust* 15–19
59 Starr, *The Social Transformation of American Medicine*, 159
60 Vogel, 41
61 Owen Sound *Times*, 13 Oct. 1894

CHAPTER 2

1 Owen Sound *Times*, 17 Oct. 1895
2 Ibid., 16 Dec. 1904
3 *Annual Report*, 1915; Owen Sound *Sun*, 25 Oct. 1912
4 OSP, 1898, no. 35, Board of Health, Report from Owen Sound for 1897; 1903, no. 36, Board of Health, Report from Owen Sound for 1902
5 Owen Sound *Times*, 16 Dec. 1904; Minutes, 2 Nov. 1906; *Annual Report*, 1908
6 Ibid.
7 Tables 2, 3, and 4 have been constructed from the admissions registers of the Owen Sound General and Marine Hospital. The total number of patients admitted annually, average length of stay, and total annual patient days may vary slightly from data reported in the Ontario Sessional Papers (Inspector of Hospitals and, later, Department of Health) which, for grant calculation purposes, treated continuing patients in residence at the start of each new fiscal year as new admissions. In order to reduce the number of missing observations, Tables 2, 3, and 4 exclude patients reportedly remaining in hospital past the end of the hospital year (Sept. 30). The diagnostic categories employed in these tables are those used by the Ontario Ministry of Health from the 1930s through the 1950s. Although they are not as refined as the widely accepted International Classification of Diseases, for the purposes of this analysis they aggregate admissions by cause into more readily understood groups.
8 See Richard H. Meade, *An Introduction to the History of General Surgery* (Toronto 1968), esp. 224–324; Public Archives of Ontario (henceforward PAO), Middlebro Papers, Biographical Sketch; Owen Sound *Daily Sun-Times*, 14 March 1930 (Frizzell Obituary)
9 See Chapter 3. The history of childbirth among modern Canadian women is discussed in Veronica Strong-Boag, *The New Day Recalled: The Lives of Girls and Women in English Canada, 1919–1939* (Toronto 1988), ch. 5, esp. 155–61.
10 See Edward Shorter, *A History of Women's Bodies* (London 1983), 143–63.
11 Minutes, 10 Feb. 1904

12 Ibid., 7 Oct. 1914; Report of Annual Inspection, 2 Oct. 1914; *Annual Report*, 1916
13 See *Annual Reports*
14 Shorter, 243–6; Meade, 155, 318
15 Minutes, 20 Feb. 1907
16 Minutes, 15 Nov. 1896, 8 Oct. 1897; 6 Dec. 1899
17 Board of Trustees' Letterbook, 1901–1930, J.M. Telford to Miss C. Sinclair, 24 July 1903; Telford to Captain McDougall, Steamer Athabaska, 31 July 1903. (Henceforward cited as Letterbook)
18 Owen Sound *Times*, 7 March, 4 April 1895
19 Minutes, 4 Oct. 1895, 11 Nov. 1898
20 Minutes, 26 Oct. 1903
21 Owen Sound *Times*, 21 Oct. 1904
22 Letterbook, Telford to J.H. Moore, 17 July 1911
23 Minutes, 9 Sept. 1914
24 Owen Sound *Sun*, 23 June 1899; Letterbook, Telford to various municipal officials, 12, 17 Sept., 21 Oct. 1902, 4 July 1903
25 These data were collated from OSP, Annual Reports of the Inspector of Prisons and Charities, 1894–1915; see Table 4.
26 Minutes, 15 Jan., 10 Feb. 1904
27 Minutes, 18 Jan., 1 Aug. 1904
28 G&M Hospital, Report of Committee to Gather Information on the Advisability of Establishing a Training School for Nurses, 12 Oct. 1900
29 Owen Sound *Times*, 22 Sept. 1911
30 Minutes, Dr T.F. Chamberlain to Dr Alan Cameron, 9 March 1903 (copy); Medical Staff to Board, 25 March 1903; *Annual Report*, 1904
31 Owen Sound *Advertiser*, 21 Nov. 1903
32 See Susan Reverby, 'The Search for the Hospital Yardstick: Nursing and the Rationalization of Hospital Work,' in *Health Care in America: Essays in Social History*, ed. Susan Reverby and David Rosner (Philadelphia 1979), 210–12.
33 See Nancy Tomes, '"Little World of Our Own": The Pennsylvania Hospital Training School for Nurses, 1895–1907,' in *Women and Health in America*, ed. Judith W. Leavitt (Madison, 1984), esp. 476–77; Judi Coburn, ' "I See and Am Silent": A Short History of Nursing in Ontario,' in *Women at Work: Ontario, 1850–1930* (Toronto 1974), esp. 140–5.
34 'The Life of a Nurse,' Toronto *Globe*, 8 Oct. 1886, in *Sara Jeanette Duncan: Selected Journalism*, ed. Thomas Tauskey (Ottawa 1978), 29
35 Owen Sound *Sun*, 31 March 1899; Minutes, 26 Aug. 1901; Owen Sound *Advertiser*, 21 Nov. 1904
36 Minutes, 23 June 1903
37 *Annual Report*, 1907; Minutes, 9 June, 8 July 1909
38 Owen Sound *Times*, 16 Dec. 1904; Minutes, 14 April, 4 May 1909
39 'Hospitals and the Medical Profession,' *Canadian Lancet*, 41 (Sept. 1907):71–2

40 Owen Sound *Times*, 12 Aug. 1904; Minutes, 2 Nov. 1906; *Annual Report*, 1907, 1908
41 Minutes, 12 Aug. 1908
42 Owen Sound *Times*, 16 Dec. 1904; Minutes, 28 April 1905, 2 Nov. 1906
43 Minutes, 2 Nov. 1906, 10 July 1907, 13 Oct. 1908, 12 May 1909
44 Minutes, 10 April 1907, 9, 23 April 1908
45 Minutes, 9 June 1909
46 Minutes, Report of Annual Meeting, 30 Nov. 1909
47 Owen Sound *Times*, 16 June 1910; Owen Sound *Sun*, 16 April 1912
48 Minutes, 30 Nov. 1909; 8 June 1910; Owen Sound *Times*, 23, 25, Aug. 1910
49 Minutes, 13 April 1910; *Annual Report*, 1909
50 Minutes, 8, 11 June 1910
51 'Subscribers to Owen Sound G&M Hospital,' *Annual Report*, 1910
52 Owen Sound *Times*, 23 June 1910; *Annual Report*, 1910; Letterbook, Telford to Grey County Council, 29 June 1913
53 Owen Sound *Times*, 6 July 1911
54 Owen Sound *Times*, 22 Sept. 1911
55 Report of Annual Inspection, 15 June 1911
56 *Annual Report*, 1912
57 *Annual Report*, 1912, 1913, 1914; Minutes, 11 Sept. 1912
58 Minutes, 21 Dec. 1910, 11 Sept. 1912, 13 Feb. 1913
59 See *Saving the Canadian City: The First Phase, 1880–1920*, ed. Paul Rutherford (Toronto 1974), Introduction.
60 *Annual Report*, 1912

CHAPTER 3

1 'Equipment of the New Toronto General Hospital,' *The Hospital World* 1 (April 1912):239–42 (henceforward *HW*)
2 OSP, 1915, no. 21, Board of Health
3 Owen Sound *Sun*, 20 June 1911; 1 April 1916
4 Edmond D. Pellegrino, 'The Sociocultural Impact of Twentieth-Century Therapeutics,' in *The Therapeutic Revolution: Essays in the Social History of American Medicine*, ed. Charles Rosenberg and Morris Vogel (Philadelphia 1979), 247–52
5 G&M Hospital, Inventory of Drugs, 30 Sept. 1931
6 Rosemary Gagan, 'Mortality Patterns and Public Health in Hamilton, Canada, 1900–1914,' *Urban History Review*, 57 (Feb., 1989):161–76
7 N.E. McKinnon, 'Mortality Reductions in Ontario, 1900–1942,' *Canadian Journal of Public Health*, 36 (July 1945):285–98
8 Owen Sound *Sun*, 1 April 1916
9 'Salutatory,' *HW* 1 (Jan. 1912):1–3; 'The Patient – A Personality, Not a Case,' ibid., 4–5
10 Ibid., 1 (May 1912):307–11

11 Ibid., 300-3
12 *Annual Report*, 1917
13 *Annual Report*, 1915
14 Minutes, 9 Dec. 1914, 13 Jan. 1915, 10 Feb. 1915, 9 May 1917
15 Minutes, 7 Oct. 1914; Report of Annual Inspection, 2 Oct. 1914, 29 Aug. 1917; *Annual Report*, 1917
16 Report of Annual Inspection, 1917
17 For a global treatment of this pandemic see Richard Collier, *The Plague of the Spanish Lady: The Influenza Epidemic of 1918-1919* (New York 1974); an American case study is Albert Crosby Jr's *Epidemic and Peace, 1918* (New Haven 1976). The impact of the epidemic on Canada is summarized in Janice P. Dickin McGinnis, 'The Impact of Epidemic Influenza, Canada, 1918-1919,' *Historical Papers* (Ottawa 1977), 120-41.
18 OSP, no. 21, 1919, Board of Health; Owen Sound *Sun*, 18, 25, 29 Oct., 1, 25 Nov., 17 Dec. 1918
19 Owen Sound *Sun-Times*, 17 Dec. 1918
20 Owen Sound *Sun*, 22 March, 2, 9 April, 10 May 1918
21 Ibid., 20 June, 25 July, 30 Oct. 1919; *Annual Report*, 1919
22 Abel-Smith, *The Hospital*, 301
23 *Annual Report*, 1915; Reports of Annual Inspection, 1917, 1919; Owen Sound *Sun*, 2 April 1918
24 *Annual Report*, 1919
25 See J.T. O'Connor, 'The Adoption and Effects of X-Rays in Ontario,' *Ontario History*, 79 (March 1987):92-107.
26 Minutes, 8 April, 28 May 1914
27 *Annual Report*, 1917; Reports of Annual Inspection, 1917; Owen Sound *Sun-Times*, 13 Dec. 1918; Minutes, 12 Feb. 1919, 14 Sept. 1922; *Annual Report*, 1922
28 Owen Sound *Sun-Times*, 17 Feb. 1923
29 Owen Sound *Daily Sun-Times*, 14 March 1930, 28 Feb. 1946, 2 Feb. 1960, 23 April 1932, 16 July 1935
30 *American Medical Directory* 1 (Chicago 1906), 26 (Chicago 1931); *The Ontario Medical Register* (Toronto 1903, 1922)
31 Rosen, 'Historical Sociology of a Community Institution,' 31
32 Owen Sound Medical Society (OSMS), Minutes, 1919-34, various entries
33 See G. Harvey Agnew, *Canadian Hospitals 1920-1970: A Dramatic Half Century* (Toronto 1974), 32-4.
34 OSMS, Minutes, 21 Jan. 1921; OSP, no. 21, 1922, Board of Health; Owen Sound *Daily Sun-Times*, 7 Jan., 11 March 1925
35 OSMS, Minutes, 6 Jan., 28 April 1922; *Annual Report*, 1922
36 *Annual Report*, 1923, 1924; Minutes, 13 Feb. 1923, 9 Dec. 1925
37 OSP, 1910-29, Registrar General's Annual Reports
38 Owen Sound *Sun-Times*, 17 Dec. 1921, 14 Feb. 1923

39 OSP, no. 14, 1927, Board of Health
40 'Ontario Hospital Association Convention,' *The Canadian Hospital* 5 (Nov. 1928):11–12
41 Barbara Melosh, 'More than "The Physician's Hand": Skill and Authority in Twentieth-Century Nursing,' in *Women and Health in America*, 482–3
42 'Hurrah, Hurrah, for Canada,' *HW* 1 (March 1912):214–16
43 OSP, no. 14, 1928, Board of Health, Division of Nurse Registration
44 Owen Sound *Sun-Times*, 19 May 1921
45 *Annual Report*, 1921, 1925; Report of Annual Inspection, 22 June 1922
46 Report of Annual Inspection, 22 June 1922
47 OSP, no. 14, 1928, Division of Nurse Registration; *Annual Report*, 1923, 1926
48 *Annual Report*, 1926
49 Minutes, 11 Feb. 1925
50 *Annual Report*, 1926; Minutes, 14 Dec. 1927
51 Owen Sound *Daily Sun-Times*, 12, 15, 19, 21, 28 Dec. 1928. Henceforward the *Daily Sun-Times* was the only regularly published newspaper in Owen Sound. To make repetitive citation of the journal less cumbersome, it is cited hereinafter as *DST*.
52 *Annual Report*, 1926, 1927
53 *DST*, 3 Jan., 21 Feb., 20 April, 8 May, 14 June 1928; Minutes, 28 April 1928
54 *Annual Report*, 1929
55 'New Owen Sound Hospital Wing,' *The Canadian Hospital* 6 (Oct. 1929):28 (henceforward *CH*); *DST*, 16 July 1929
56 Ibid.; *DST*, 16 July 1929; *Annual Report*, 1929
57 *Annual Report*, 1929
58 'More Publicity Is Needed,' *CH* 5 (Sept. 1928):11; 'Is the Public out of Touch with the Hospital?' *CH* 6 (July 1929):11
59 'Ontario Hospital Association Convention,' *CH* 5 (Nov. 1928):11
60 'Paying the Hospital Bill,' *CH* 4 (Nov. 1927):9
61 'Latest Hospital Report Shows Charges Are 90 Per Cent Higher,' *CH* 6 (Dec. 1929):31
62 Hospitals Handicapped by Meagre Grants,' *CH* 4 (Nov. 1927):11–12
63 *DST*, 18 July 1929
64 Ibid., 24 Sept. 1956
65 *Annual Report*, 1929
66 Charles Rosenberg, 'The Therapeutic Revolution: Medicine, Meaning and Social Change in Nineteenth-Century America,' in *The Therapeutic Revolution*, 15

CHAPTER 4

1 *DST*, 27 Jan. 1933, 2 Jan. 1937

Notes to pp. 85–93   151

2  Michiel Horn, ed., *The Dirty Thirties* (Toronto 1972), 12; see H. Blair Neatby, *The Politics of Chaos* (Toronto 1972), esp. ch. 2.
3  Province of Ontario, Department of Health, Division of Medical Statistics, *A Survey of Public General Hospitals in Ontario*, Part 1 (Toronto 1940), 20–5
4  'A Hospital Problem Survey,' *CH* 3 (Feb. 1926):12; 'Hospitals Handicapped by Meagre Grants,' *CH*, 4 (Nov. 1927):11–12; 'Representative Deputation Presses Claims at Parliament Buildings,' *CH* 5 (Feb. 1928):14
5  See C. David Naylor, *Private Practice, Public Payment: Canadian Medicine and the Politics of Health Insurance, 1911–1956* (Montreal 1986), 35–41.
6  'The Care of the Sick,' *Canadian Medical Association Journal* 17 (Jan. 1927):94–7 (henceforward, *CMAJ*)
7  James McKenty, 'The Relations of the Medical Profession to Hospitals,' *CMAJ* 17 (Feb. 1927):151-2
8  Province of Ontario, Department of Health, *The Hospitals of Ontario: A Short History* (Toronto 1934), 20
9  Province of Ontario, Royal Commission on Public Welfare, *Report* (Toronto 1930), 14–15
10  H.H. Robbins (Deputy Provincial Secretary), 'Address Delivered before the Ontario Hospital Association,' *Canadian Lancet* 77 (4, 1931):105–10
11  *DST*, 25, 27 Jan., 11 Sept., 14 Oct. 1930
12  Ibid., 15 Nov., 13 Dec. 1930
13  Ibid., 26 July, 8 Aug. 1931
14  Ibid., 7 Oct. 1931
15  Ibid., 16 Oct. 1930, Government of Canada, Census of Institutions, 1931, 'Owen Sound General and Marine Hospital' (file copy)
16  OSMS, Minutes, 24 Oct. 1930; *DST*, 26 Aug., 28 Sept. 1930; 2 Feb. 1931
17  Ibid., 23 Oct. 1931; data cited are drawn from OSP, Inspector of Hospitals, Annual Reports.
18  Ibid., 15 May 1936
19  OSMS, Minutes, 10 Jan., 28 July 1933; OSMS, Correspondence, G.W. McQuay (City Finance Committee) to Miss B. Hall, superintendent, G&M Hospital, 29 April 1933 (copy) and G.W. McQuay to OSMS, 13 May 1933; *DST*, 27 Jan., 19, 27 Feb., 11 March 1933
20  *DST*, 25 Oct. 1936
21  Minutes, 10 Feb., 13 April, 14 July, 8 Aug. 1932; *DST*, 16 Jan. 1934
22  *DST*, 16 Jan., 15 Feb. 1934
23  OSMS, Minutes, 7 Oct. 1932, 12 Oct. 1934; OSMS, Correspondence, F.C. Routley to G. Morris, 11 Oct. 1932; H.W. Aikens to S.E. Morris, 16 Nov. 1936; *DST*, 28 June 1934
24  G&M Hospital, Miscellaneous Correspondence, Bertha Hall to Miss A. Munn (Inspector of Nurses' Training Schools), 10 June 1932; board of trustees to A. Munn, 7 Nov. 1932

25 Grey County Museum, G&M School of Nursing Files, Report of Inspection on Nurses' Training School, 12 June 1933 (henceforward GMSN)
26 *DST*, 18 Oct. 1933
27 Ibid., GMSN, Report of Inspection, 28 Aug. 1934
28 GMSN, Report of Inspection, 15 Dec. 1935 and (undated) 1937
29 *DST*, 1 Oct. 1930
30 Minutes, 14, 21 May, 1 June, 12 Aug., 11 Dec. 1936; 5, 15 Jan. 1937; *DST*, 18 Dec. 1936, 6 Jan. 1937
31 *DST*, 11 Feb. 1932; 9 July 1933; 6 April 1935; 2 May 1936; Minutes, 13 May 1937
32 Minutes, 6 June, 11 Aug. 1938; *DST*, 15 Oct., 11 Nov. 1938
33 *DST*, 3, 11 March 1939
34 Ibid., 23 March 1939
35 Ibid., 15 Oct. 1938, 23 March 1939
36 OSMS, Minutes, 27 Jan. 1939; *DST*, 24 Feb. 1940
37 'Health Insurance Survey Completed by McGill Expert,' *CH* 9 (June 1932):11
38 'The Proposed Hospital Care Plan for Ontario,' *CH* 16 (June 1939):28
39 *A Survey of Public General Hospitals in Ontario*, Part 1, summary
40 G&M Hospital, Miscellaneous Reports, Superintendent's Report re Training School, July 1940
41 *DST*, 3 Feb. 1941
42 Ibid., 5 Feb. 1943, 11 Feb. 1944
43 Minutes, Feb.–Sept. 1942; *DST*, 6 Feb. 1942
44 *DST*, 14 June 1941, 11 Oct. 1946
45 OSMS, minutes, 29 March 1940
46 Ibid., 11 Feb. 1944
47 Minutes, 13 Nov. 1941, 14 Oct. 1943; see 'Public Relations,' *CH* 14 (Oct. 1937):64
48 Minutes, 22 March 1943, 6 March 1944, 30 July 1944; 'Brief to ... the Mayor and Aldermen of the City of Owen Sound' (1943)
49 Minutes, 15 Feb. 1945, containing copy of letter, C.A. Eberle to James Garvie, 18 Dec. 1944
50 Minutes, Jan.–Dec. 1945; *DST*, 22 Feb. 1946
51 Ibid.
52 Minutes, March–May 1946, 10 April 1947
53 See, e.g., *CH* 17 (May 1940):27; *The Hospital in Modern Society*, ed. Arthur C. Bachmeyer and Gerhard Hartman (New York 1943).
54 Minutes, 22 June 1946
55 'Aid to Ontario Hospitals on Basis of Public Ward Beds,' *CH* 24 (April 1947): 25; Minutes, 7 May 1947
56 *DST*, 6 May 1933
57 *DST*, 10 June, 25 Sept., 27 Nov. 1947
58 Ibid., 15 Aug., 5 Sept. 1947; Minutes, 11 Oct. 1948. Total cost of reconstructing and refurbishing the hut as a residence was $45,000.

59 Public Archives of Ontario (PAO), Ministry of Health, OHSC, Central Files, Department of Health, C.J. Telfer to J.T. Phair, 16 June 1949
60 Malcolm G. Taylor, *Health Insurance and Canadian Public Policy: The Seven Decisions That Created the Canadian Health Insurance System* (Montreal 1978), 54; Naylor, *Private Practice*, 163-84

CHAPTER 5

1 Canada, House of Commons, Special Committee on Social Security, *Health Insurance: Report of the Advisory Committee on Health Insurance* (Ottawa 1943)
2 Canada, House of Commons, Special Committee on Social Security, Minutes of Proceedings and Evidence (6, 9 April 1943), 174-5
3 Canada, House of Commons, Special Committee on Social Security, L.C. Marsh, *Report on Social Security for Canada* (Ottawa 1943), 55
4 Malcolm G. Taylor, *Health Insurance* 2-3
5 J.E.F. Hastings, 'Federal-Provincial Insurance for Hospital and Physician's Care in Canada,' *International Journal of Health Services* 1 (1971): 401
6 Province of Ontario, Ministry of Health, *Report of the Ontario Health Survey Committee* 1 (Toronto 1950): 23, Table A7; Canada, Department of National Health and Welfare, *Hospital Care in Canada: Recent Trends and Developments*, Health Care Series, Memorandum no. 12 (Ottawa 1960), 77-8
7 Dominion Bureau of Statistics, *Canadian Sickness Survey, 1950-51*, Special Compilation No. 1, *Family Expenditures for Health Services* (Ottawa 1953), Tables 1-2
8 *DST*, 10 April 1950; G&M Hospital, Miscellaneous Reports, Report of the Medical staff for 1949 (undated, 1950)
9 Minutes, 22 Feb. 1951
10 PAO, OHSC Central Files, Ontario Department of Health, M.J. Stalker to File, 20 July 1950
11 *DST*, 17 Feb. 1950; *Hospital Care in Canada* 46-58
12 These data can be compared with those compiled by the Department of National Health and Welfare which indicate similar national trends, although the growth of graduate nursing staff nationally was slower. One reason for the difference between the national and the Owen Sound data is that the latter represent both full- and part-time salaried nurses. See *Hospital Care in Canada*, 50.
13 Minutes, Annual Report for 1952
14 Minutes, Finance Committee Report, 10 Dec. 1945
15 These data are calculated from the G&M's financial report for 1951 as reported in *DST*, 22 Feb. 1952.
16 *Hospital Care in Canada*, 75
17 *DST*, 22 March 1950
18 *Report of the Ontario Hospital Survey Committee*, 1:26. The foregoing summary is

drawn from the overview presented in Chapters 1 and 2 and Table A54 of Vol. 1 of the report.
19 *DST*, 23 Feb. 1950
20 *DST*, 17 Feb. 5 May 1950
21 Ibid., 14 April 1948
22 Ibid., 23 Oct. 1950
23 PAO, OHSC, Central Files, Department of Health, Application for a Capital Grant for Hospital Construction, Owen Sound General and Marine Hospital, 15 Aug. 1950
24 *DST*, 21 Nov. 1950
25 Ibid., 2 Jan. 1951
26 Ibid., 20 April, 6, 15 June 1951
27 Ibid., 13 June, 22 Sept. 21 Oct. 1952
28 Ibid., 14 Dec. 1952
29 Minutes, 16 April, 18 June 1953
30 *DST*, 13, 22 Oct., 6 Nov. 1953
31 Minutes, 21 Jan., 23 Feb. 1954; *DST*, 2, 20, 29 Jan. 1954
32 Markdale *Standard*, Durham *Chronicle*, and Hanover *Post*, quoted in *DST*, 1 March 1954
33 Kincardine *News*, 8 July 1954; Chesley *Enterprise*, 12 Aug. 1954
34 *DST*, 4 Feb., 10 April, 10 May 1954
35 Ibid., 11–19 Nov. 1954
36 Ibid., 22 Jan., 23 April 1955
37 Minutes, 19 May 1955
38 Ibid., 7 Oct. 1955; 4 July, 11 Aug. 1956
39 Taylor, *Health Insurance and Canadian Public Policy*, 106–16
40 Dominion Bureau of Statistics, *Hospital Expenditures, 1959* (Ottawa 1962), Table 1; *Hospital Expenditures, 1960* (Ottawa 1960), Graph 3
41 Taylor, 116, 136–45
42 *DST*, 4 April 1957, 30 April, 25 June 1958
43 Ibid., 17 May, 25 June, 22 July, 1958; Minutes, 19 June, 17 July, 1958, 21 May 1959
44 Minutes, 21 May 1959; *DST*, 26 June 1959
45 *DST*, 19 Feb. 1960
46 *Hospital Care in Canada*, 65
47 Ibid., 18 Dec. 1959, 31 May, 30 Sept., 28 Oct., 15 Nov. 1960
48 Minutes, Annual Report for 1963 (undated 1964)
49 Canada, Department of National Health and Welfare, *Hospital Care in Canada: Trends and Development, 1948–1962*, Health Care Series, Memorandum no. 19 (Ottawa 1964), 8–9, 14–15
50 *Hospital Care in Canada*, Memorandum no. 12, 50–3. James E. Bennett and Jacques Krasny, 'Health Care in Canada,' in *Health and Canadian Society*, ed. David Coburn, Carl D'arcy, Peter New, and George Torrance (Toronto 1981),

p. 60, describe this as a phenomenon of the 1970s; but in one remarkable year, 1961, the number of outpatients treated at the G&M was 7857, 60 per cent of all patients treated.
51 *DST*, 1, 16 Jan. 1959
52 *Hospital Care in Canada*, no. 19, 57
53 *DST*, 30 April 1953
54 Lee Soderstrom, *The Canadian Health Care System* (London 1978), 161
55 Minutes, 18 Nov. 1964, 20 Jan. 1966
56 Ibid., 21 Sept. 1967
57 Ibid., 20 Oct. 1966, 17 Nov. 1966; Soderstrom, 89
58 Minutes, 27 March, 22 May 1969
59 Ibid., 8 Oct., 18 Dec. 1969, 1 July 1970
60 A decade later the provincial government's Select Committee on Health Care Financing and Costs accepted this principle as the underlying premise of health care in Ontario. See its *Report*, 17 Oct. 1978, p. 37.

CHAPTER 6

1 Gary D. Chatfield, 'The Economics of Health Care Delivery,' *Health Care Delivery Systems in North America: The Changing Concepts* (Windsor 1977), 83–5
2 Province of Ontario, Legislature, Select Committee on Health Care Financing and Costs, *Report*, 1978, 14–15
3 Bennett and Krasny, 'Health Care in Canada,' 46–56
4 Pellegrino, 'The Sociocultural Impact of Twentieth-Century Therapeutics,' 246
5 G&M Admissions and Discharge Committee, *Report*, Dec. 1972; Minutes, 29 Sept. 1974, 15 May, 24 Sept, 20 Nov. 1975
6 Andrew Armitage, 'Smallpox Epidemics Led to Drive for First Hospital,' *DST*, 6 March 1976
7 Minutes, 16 Nov. 1967
8 Ibid., 1 April, 17 June, 1971, 20 Jan. 1972
9 Ibid., 21 Dec. 1972, 24 Jan., 30 May, 20 June 1974
10 Stephen Storcz, 'Community Health Services: A Return to Neighbourhood,' in *Health Care Delivery Systems in North America*, 126–7; Minutes, 24 Jan. 1974
11 *DST*, 30 Oct. 1979
12 Ibid., Minutes, 9 Jan. 1978

# Index

Act to Establish the Hospital Services Commission of Ontario (1958), 121
American College of Surgeons, 71
Antisepsis, 12, 49, 61
Armitage, Andrew, 155 n.6
Asepsis, 12, 61
Associated Medical Services, Inc., 98, 111

Barnhart, Dr Charles, 15
Berlin (Kitchener), 7
Beveridge, Sir William, 110
Blue Cross, 111
Board of Health (Ontario), 8, 71
Boosterism, 7, 11
Brantford, 7, 18
Brewster, Dr F.A., 69
Brown, Reta, 105
Bruce County, 5; Council, 117, 119–20
Busy Bees, 3
Butchart, D.M., 53, 76, 81

Cameron, Dr Allan, 9–10, 15–16, 18
*Canadian Co-operator and Patron, The*, 8
*Canadian Hospital, The*, 77–8
Canadian Hospital Association, 60
Canadian Hospital Council, 110

*Canadian Lancet*, 15, 49
Canadian Medical Association, 99; and care of indigents, 86
Canadian Pacific Railway, 4–5; steamships, 5–6
Canadian Sickness Survey (1950), 111
Case, Garfield, 104
Chamberlain, Dr F., 19, 21, 23
Charity Aid Act (1874), 14, 19
Chatham, 4
Chatsworth, 16
Chesley, 134
Christie and Agee, 18
Clark, James, 105
Collingwood, 5
Creasor, Alfred, 81

Danard, Dr A.L., 69–70, 111
Davis, Hon. William, 132
Department of Health (Ontario). *See* Ministry of Health
Department of National Health and Welfare (Canada), 114
Derby Township, 37, 53
Detroit Children's Hospital, 94
District health councils, 133–4
Dominion Grange, 8

Dominion Grange Mutual Insurance Company, 8
Dominion Lands Act (1870), 5
Dow, Dr W. George, 16, 21, 69-70
Doyle, R.J., 8
Drew, Hon. George, 107, 111
Duncan, Jessie, 50, 59
Duncan, Sara Jeanette, 47
Duplessis, Maurice, 111
Durham, 119, 134

Eberle, C.A., 104
Electric Illumination and Manufacturing Company (Owen Sound), 7, 16, 79
Evans, Dr E.E., 69

Family: and medical care, 28
Freemasons, 3
French, Dr Gordon, 96
Frizzell, Dr W.T., 35, 69-70
Frost, Mayor John, 3
Frost, Hon. Leslie, 106, 121

Galt, 7, 18
Gaviller, Dr Charles, 69
General and Marine Hospital
- accessibility, 30, 33, 34, 77, 112, 118, 127
- accounts in arrears, 43
- administrative structure, 20, 139
- administrators, list of, 141
- admissions, 30, 73, 76, 88, 90, 101-2, 123, 126, 132; geographical distribution, 37; indigent patients, 23, 29, 38, 91, 114; obstetric, 36, 68; paying patients, 24, 32, 38, 50; by sex, 37-8; surgical, 36, 68
- Board of Governors, 16, 26; executive, 105 (continuity, 79-81; presidents, list of, 142; structure of, 104-5); Building and Grounds Committee, 26; House Committee, 17, 26, 43; Public Relations Committee, 104
- construction costs (1893), 18
- debts, 54, 77, 96
- deficits, 51, 91-2, 104, 116, 132
- departments, 105, 111, 125; ambulance, 72; cardiology, 125; chronic care, 126, 127; laboratory, 71, 96, 132-3; medical records, 96; nuclear medicine, 133; obstetrics, 50, 66, 76, 102; outpatients, 125, 126, 129; pathology, 71; pediatrics, 126; pharmacy, 132-3; physiotherapy, 125; radiology, 68-9, 96, 102, 132; surgery, 132
- fees, 40, 54, 88
- fund-raising, 16, 19, 41, 52-3, 67, 76, 78, 106, 134
- infant mortality, 102
- medical staff, 19-20, 24, 69, 101, 138; and criticism of Matron, 20-1, 49, 95; and hospital modernization, 49-50; morbidity (1920s), 32-5, 82-3, 99-100
- motto, 18
- and national health insurance, 129-30
- operating costs, 41, 45, 81-2, 102, 113; wages, 51, 112-13, 128
- origins, 10
- patient stays, 32-3, 90, 126
- physical plant, 18, 58; expansion, 50-3, 77, 106, 117, 120, 122-3, 127, 134; laundry, 48, 68; lighting, 48; morgue, 68; refrigeration, 48, 68, 96
- public relations, 121
- purchasing policies, 45-6
- revenues, 39-40, 90, 102, 113, 114, 123, 125; collection boxes, 42; in kind, 42-3; municipal grants, 43-4; subscriptions, 41; subsidies, government, 45, 55; surcharges, 50, 107, 119
- *Rules and Regulations*, 20, 25

– School of Nursing: admissions standards, 75, 95; curriculum, 47, 75, 94; living conditions, 74–5; origins, 46–7; recruitment (1940s), 101; residence, 51, 93–4, 101, 107, 123; transfer to Georgian College, 128
– site, 16, 17–18, 128
– standardization, 70–2
– workforce, 23, 46, 54, 101, 112–13, 128, 132; certification, 113; staff/patient ratios, 112–13
Government of Ontario: grants to hospitals, 19, 61–3, 79, 85–7; health care costs, 132; Inspector of Prisons and Charities, 22
Grand Trunk Railway, 7
Gray, Dr Eliza, 23
Great Depression: effect on national health, 84–5
Greene, Alex, 18
'Greys, The' (147/248 Battalions), 66
Grey-Bruce Health Services Planning Commission. *See* district health councils
Grey Bruce Regional Health Centre, 135
Grey County, 5, 37: Council, 16, 44, 106–7, 116–20; population, 37, 71
Guelph, 7

Hall, Bertha, 95
Hanover, 119, 134
Harrison, E.J., 81
Harrison, F.W., 63, 81
Harrison, John, 16, 76
Heagerty Committee, 110
Hipwell, Norval, 120
Holmes, Dr G.W., 81, 95, 97–8
Hospital Day, 43
Hospital Insurance and Diagnostic Services Act (Canada, 1958), 122
*Hospital World*, 60, 62
Hospitals: accessibility, 29, 122;

administration, 12, 22, 60, 106; history, nineteenth century, 11–14; history, Ontario, 14; and care of indigents, 85, 108, 115; morbidity and mortality (Ontario), 14; municipal subsidies, 115; operating costs, 121; patient stays, 115; provincial subsidies, 115; revenue, 61–3, 99; and social classes, 13; and surgical revolution, 28; therapeutic effectiveness, 59; transformation of (1900–20), 29; volume of care delivered, 125
Hospitals and Charitable Institutions Act (1912), 61–2, 75, 87
Howey, Dr Richard, 35, 69–70

Imperial Order Daughters of the Empire, 75
Inglis Falls, 7
Insurance: national health, 98, 108, 110, 121, 129–30; voluntary group health insurance, 98, 111

James, John, 69

Kelley, Hon. Russell T., 116
Kelso, J.J., 8
Keppel Township, 37
Kilbourn, J.M., 16, 53
Kincardine, 134
King, Hon. William Lyon Mackenzie, 101, 104, 110, 121
King's Daughters, 3
Knox (Presbyterian) Church, 7

Ladies' Auxiliary. *See* Women's Auxiliary
Ladies' Hospital Aid. *See* Women's Auxiliary
Lady superintendent(s), 12, 23, 105–6; list of, 141
Lediard, Rev. John, 8

Lemon, Mrs Elias, 81
LePan, Frederic d'Orr, 16
Lion's Head, 134
Listerism. *See* asepsis; antisepsis
Little, R.D., 81

McArthur, Jennie, 81
McCullough, Dr James, 15
Mackinnon Phillips Psychiatric Hospital, 133, 135
McLinden, Joseph R., 79, 91, 95
MacNaughton, Gen. A.G.L., 104
Markdale, 119
Meaford, 119
Medical Care Act (Canada, 1966), 126
Middlebro, Dr T.H., 35, 52, 69–70
Miller, Hon. Frank, 132
Ministry of Health (Ontario), 99, 107, 116, 118, 122
Moore, J.E. (matron), 20–1
Mount Forest, 119, 134
Mulock, Sir William, 76

National Health Grants Program (Canada), 111–12
Nightingale, Florence, 12, 22
Nurse Registration Act (Ontario, 1922), 75
Nurses: and hospital management, 22–3; opportunities for (1920s), 73; professionalization (1890s), 47; registration (Ontario), 62

Ontario, Province of: social and economic development, 4
Ontario College of Physicians and Surgeons, 93
Ontario Health Survey (1950), 115
Ontario Health Survey Committee, 121
Ontario Hospital (London), 95
Ontario Hospital Association, 73, 85–6, 98

Ontario Hospital Insurance Plan, 123
Ontario Hospital Services Commission, 128, 132–3
Ontario Municipal Board, 118
Owen Sound
- Collegiate Institute, 7
- Council, Town (City), 10, 16–17, 44, 96–7, 116–17
- early history, 3–8
- economic development, 4–5
- Hospital Debenture Referendum, 117–18
- medical relief (1930s), 90, 98
- medical relief officers, 91–2
- mortality rates, 9
- population, 4–6, 71, 109
- public health, 8–10; child welfare clinic, 71; communicable diseases, 9, 30, 75–6; municipal water supply, 7, 71; Spanish Influenza (1918), 66–7; tuberculosis, 34, 75; typhoid fever, 30, 34, 66
- public libraries, 7
- taverns, 6
- transients, 6
- unemployment relief, 87–8, 92
- Welfare Board, 88, 92
Owen Sound General and Marine Hospital Trust: incorporation, 145 n.42; membership, 17, 26
Owen Sound and Grey and Bruce Loan and Savings Company, 16, 49
Owen Sound Medical Society, 70, 90, 97–8

Parker, John, 81
Parker, S.J., 16, 19
Paterson, Roland, 67
Paterson House Hotel, 7
Patients: indigent, 13, 100, 108; paying, 13, 78–9, 100; and therapeutic revolution, 109

Penicillin, 102
Perth, 4
Phillips, Dr Mackinnon, 114, 116, 118, 121
Physicians: and irregular practitioners, 15; and medical professionalism, 15, 21, 28; and 'scientific' medicine, 12
Prince Arthur's Landing, 5
Public Hospitals Act (1931), 87

Redmond, Margaret, 81
Rockefeller, John D., 52–3
Roy, William, 16
Royal Commission on Public Welfare (Ontario, 1930), 87
Royal Loan and Savings Company (Brantford), 16
Rutherford, Dr A.B., 69–70

St. George's (Anglican) Church, 7
Sarawak Township, 15, 37
Sargent, Mayor E.C., 118, 120
Sarnia, 4
Select Committee on Health Care Financing and Costs (Ontario, 1978), 131
Smith, W.H., 51
Southampton, 134
Special Committee on Social Security (Canada), 110
Standardization movement, 70
Stirling, Maude, 81
Stratford, 7, 18
Streptomycin, 102
Sullivan Township, 37
*Sun* (Owen Sound), 67

*Sun-Times* (Owen Sound), 67, 69, 74, 88, 98, 116
*Survey of Public General Hospitals in Ontario* (1940), 99
Sydenham Township, 37, 53

Telford, Col. J.P., 43
Thompson, Georgina, 81
*Times* (Owen Sound), 6, 7, 9, 17, 19, 42, 53
Tolton, John, 26
Toronto, 7
Toronto General Hospital, 10, 14, 57
Toronto Grey and Bruce Railway, 5
Tuberculosis, 34, 59, 75
Typhoid fever, 9–10, 30, 34, 66

University of Toronto, 14, 70

Vivian, Hon. R.P., 104
Voluntarism, 13, 22, 139

Walkerton, 134
War Assets Disposal Corporation, 107
Webb, Dr Gordon, 82, 92–3
Wiarton, 53, 134
Widdifield, Judge, 67
Woman's Christian Temperance Union, 7
Woman's Missionary Society (Methodist Church of Canada), 8
Women's Auxiliary (G&M), 16, 17, 19, 36, 43, 48, 51, 68, 76, 94
Woods, Ethel, 81

X-rays, 12, 68–9